Patient Teaching Guides for Health Promotion

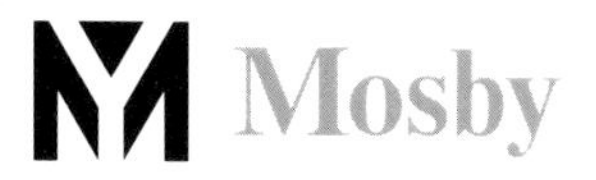

St. Louis Baltimore Boston Carlsbad Chicago Naples New York Philadelphia Portland
London Madrid Mexico City Singapore Sydney Tokyo Toronto Wiesbaden

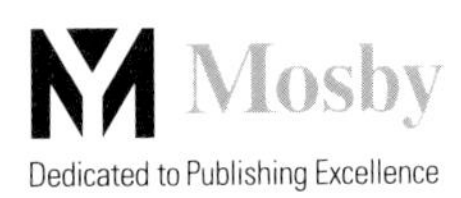

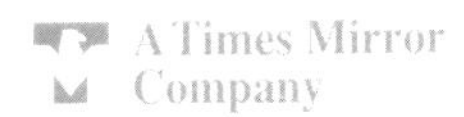

Vice-President and Publisher: Nancy L. Coon
Senior Editor: Sally Schrefer
Developmental Editor: Gail Brower
Project Manager: Mark Spann
Designer: Judi Lang
Manufacturing Manager: Betty Mueller

Printed in the United States of America

Composition by The Clarinda Company
Printing/binding by Mulligan Printing Co.

Mosby–Year Book, Inc.
11830 Westline Industrial Drive
St. Louis, Missouri 63146

ISBN 0-8151-2574-7

97 98 99 00 / 9 8 7 6 5 4 3 2 1

Cardiovascular Disease Risk Factors

Many deaths from cardiovascular disease are preventable. In addition, for people who already have been diagnosed with cardiovascular disease, the risk of death and further complications can be reduced. Research has uncovered several factors that contribute to heart attacks and strokes. The more risk factors a person has, the greater the chance of developing cardiovascular disease. Although some risk factors cannot be changed, you can modify others with your doctor's help, and still others can be eliminated altogether. The following checklists can help you determine your risk.

Major risk factors that cannot be changed

Heredity. A tendency toward heart disease runs in families. If one or both parents had cardiovascular disease, one's chances of developing it are higher.

Race. For reasons presently unknown, blacks have a much greater risk of developing high blood pressure than whites; twice as many have moderately high blood pressure, and three times as many have extremely high blood pressure. As a result, their risk of heart disease is greater.

Sex. Men have a higher risk of heart attack and stroke than women. During the childbearing years, women produce hormones that keep blood cholesterol levels low. Male hormones have the opposite effect—they raise blood cholesterol. However, women lose this protection after menopause or surgical removal of the ovaries, and women over age 55 have a 10 times greater risk than younger women. In recent years, however, more women under age 40 have developed coronary artery disease and high blood pressure. This probably results from the use of oral contraceptives and increased smoking.

Age. Fifty-five percent of heart attacks occur in people age 65 or older.

Major risk factors that can be changed

Smoking. Smokers have more than twice as many heart attacks as nonsmokers. Sudden cardiac death occurs two to four times more frequently in smokers. Peripheral vascular disease (narrowing of the blood vessels in the arms and legs) is almost exclusively a disease of smokers. When people stop smoking, the risk of heart disease drops rapidly, and 10 years after quitting, their risk of death from cardiovascular disease is about the same as for people who never smoked.

High Blood Pressure. High Blood pressure makes the heart work harder, causing it to enlarge and become weaker over time. This can lead to stroke, heart attack, kidney failure, and congestive heart failure. For some people, high blood pressure can be controlled by a low-salt diet, weight reduction, and regular exercise. Other people also require medication to lower their blood pressure.

Blood Cholesterol Levels. A cholesterol level between 200 and 240 mg/dl increases the risk of heart disease. A cholesterol level greater than 240 mg/dl doubles the risk of coronary artery disease. The American Heart Association Diet, which is low in cholesterol and other fats, is recommended for anyone with a level of 200 or higher. Medication may also be necessary.

Other risk factors

Diabetes. Diabetes increases the risk of heart attack because it raises blood cholesterol levels. In adddition, people who develop diabetes in midlife are often overweight, which is an additional risk factor.

Obesity. Excess weight forces the heart to work harder. People who are overweight are more prone to high blood pressure and high blood cholesterol levels. Obesity is defined as 30% or more over your ideal weight.

Physical Inactivity. Researchers have found that people who seldom exercise do not recover as well from heart attacks. Although it is not clear if lack of exercise alone is a risk factor for developing heart disease, in combination with other risk factors, such as overweight, the risk is higher.

Stress. Excessive emotional stress over a prolonged period appears to increase the risk of heart disease. Stress can increase other existing risk factors, such as overeating, smoking, and high blood pressure.

Oral contraceptives. Birth control pills can worsen other risk factors. They raise blood cholesterol levels and increase blood pressure, so women who already have these problems should not take oral contraceptives. Smokers who take "the pill" run the risk of developing dangerous blood clots (thrombosis).

Alcohol. Heavy drinking can cause high blood pressure and lead to heart failure. Alcohol should be consumed only in moderate amounts—2 ounces of liquor a day or less.

Controlling Your Blood Pressure

At present there is no cure for high blood pressure, but it can be controlled to reduce the chances of developing problems. This takes a team effort, and you are the most important member of the team. Mild or moderate high blood pressure can often be controlled successfully by a low-salt diet, exercise, and weight loss.

Sodium (salt) causes your body to retain fluids, which can put extra strain on the heart and make the blood vessels narrow. For this reason, low-sodium diets are recommended to reduce the amount of retained water, which then helps to lower the blood pressure. Foods that are high in potassium and calcium also help lower blood pressure.

A moderate amount of regular exercise has several benefits. It improves your overall physical conditioning, helps with weight loss by burning extra calories, reduces blood cholesterol, and may have a more direct effect on lowering your blood pressure.

Maintaining yourself at the right weight for your height and bone structure is important. Extra fat makes your heart work harder. A low-fat, low-calorie diet has the further advantage of reducing your blood cholesterol levels and delaying the beginning of arteriosclerosis. People with high blood pressure can consume moderate amounts of alcohol (about two drinks per day), but a heavy intake of alcohol raises blood pressure. If you are on a weight reduction diet, keep in mind that alcohol is high in calories.

Although high blood pressure is not caused by "bad nerves," prolonged stress does increase blood pressure. Learning to relax and taking time out to do things you enjoy should be part of your blood pressure control program.

Medication

Medication is necessary if you have severe high blood pressure or high blood pressure that is not controlled by diet, exercise, and weight reduction. Diuretics (water pills) are often prescribed to eliminate the excess sodium from your body. If diuretic therapy is not effective in bringing your blood pressure down, your doctor will add other medication to the treatment program.

Several different types of antihypertensive drugs are available: nerve blockers, beta blockers, blood vessel dilators, hormone inhibitors, and calcium channel blockers. Each type of drug works differently, but basically they control blood pressure by relaxing and opening up narrowed blood vessels. Since everyone is different, your doctor may have to try more than one drug to find the most effective medication with the fewest side effects. When your doctor prescribes an antihypertensive drug, ask about the type and possible side effects.

Be sure to keep appointments with your doctor. Several visits may be necessary to determine exactly the right drug and dosage. Once your blood pressure is under control, you will need to see your doctor only about three or four times a year.

Remember: Diuretics and antihypertensive medications lower your blood pressure only while you are taking them. You cannot stop taking the drug, even after your blood pressure is lowered.

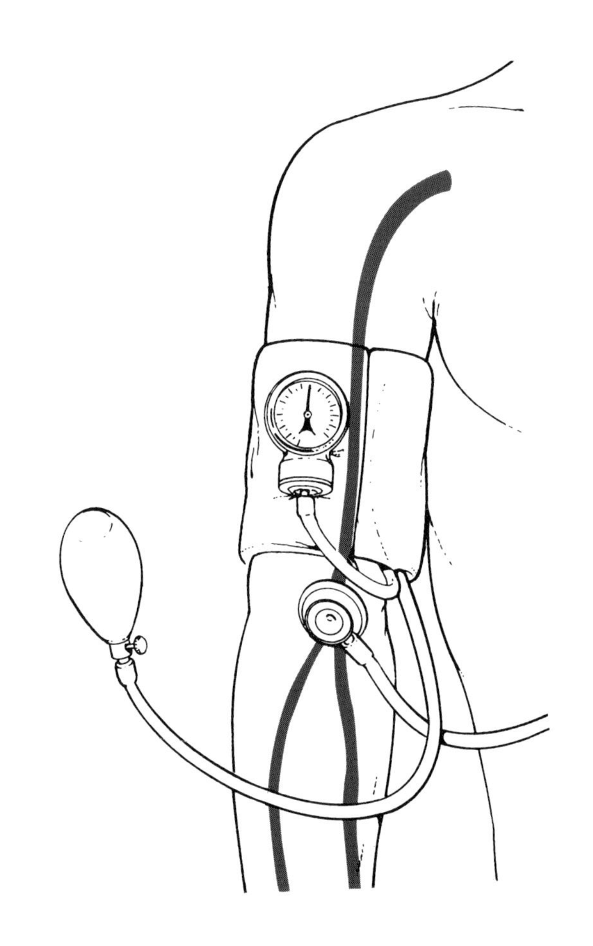

What is Cholesterol?

Cholesterol is a soft, fatlike substance, found in all cells of the body. It is needed in small quantities to keep the body healthy. When there is too much cholesterol, it may collect and lead to hardening of the arteries and heart disease or a heart attack. The amount of cholesterol in your body is determined by heredity and, in part, by diet.

Daily diets that are high in saturated fats, such as those including eggs, cheese, and fatty meats, can raise the blood cholesterol level and are associated with an increased risk of heart disease.

Types of Cholesterol

The body makes three types of cholesterol called *lipoproteins*. These are: **VLDL** (very low-density lipoproteins), **LDL** (low-density lipoproteins), and **HDL** (high-density lipoproteins).

> **VLDL** carries fat from the liver to other parts of the body. VLDL becomes LDL after it unloads fat.
>
> **LDL** is necessary for health but is often called "BAD" cholesterol because it easily becomes stuck to the side walls of the blood vessels.
>
> **HDL** is called *"GOOD"* cholesterol because it finds and unsticks LDL pieces and brings them back to the liver. HDL is good for people who eat a lot of fat in their diet.

Where Does Cholesterol Come From?

Cholesterol is not fat, but it is closely related to fats. It is a chemical that is an important part of the cells of the body and is involved in the formation of important hormones. Even if your diet contained no cholesterol, your liver would still produce all of the cholesterol your body needs. The liver makes most of your body's natural cholesterol. If you eat too much fat, your body makes more cholesterol (VLDL) to carry the fat. When this happens, more LDL becomes stuck in the blood vessels and there is not enough HDL to rescue them. When this occurs, the blood vessels may become blocked, or hardened. This is called arteriosclerosis, which may lead to an increased risk of a heart attack or other heart disease.

Cholesterol Testing

It is important to test your cholesterol at least once each year. Once you know your cholesterol levels, then you know if you are at an increased risk for heart disease. You will also know if you need to make changes in your diet to lower the cholesterol. The cholesterol test should provide three numbers: the total cholesterol, the HDL, and the LDL. Your goal should be to keep all of the numbers in the *desirable* level.

The cholesterol/HDL ratio gives more information than either HDL or cholesterol alone. The higher the cholesterol/HDL ratio, the greater the risk for developing hardening of the arteries (atherosclerosis). The table below shows the ratio risks.

What to Do If Your Cholesterol is High

If your levels fall in the *borderline* or *danger* levels, talk with your health care provider to learn ways to lower your cholesterol, such as changing your diet, exercising, and reducing other health risks like smoking, high blood pressure, and stress.

It is important that you visit your health care provider periodically to be sure that your cholesterol level is under control. If your cholesterol cannot be controlled by diet, exercise, and other lifestyle changes, it may be necessary to take a prescribed medication to help control your cholesterol.

CHOLESTEROL LEVELS

	Desirable	*Borderline*	*Danger*
TOTAL	Less than 200 mg/dl*	200 - 239 mg/dl	240 mg/dl or higher
HDL	35 mg/dl or higher	------------	Less than 35 mg/dl
LDL	Less than 130 mg/dl	130 - 159 mg/dl	160 mg/dl or higher

(* mg/dl means milligrams per deciliter [100 milliters])

CHOLESTEROL/HDL RATIO

Risk Level for Heart Disease	*Men*	*Women*
Low	3.43	3.27
Average	4.97	4.44
Moderate	9.55	7.05
High	23.99	11.04

Eating a Low-fat Diet

A low-fat diet may be recommended for several reasons, including moderately high cholesterol or dangerously high cholesterol levels over 240 mg/dl. The amount and type of fat in the diet will affect the cholesterol level in the body. Certain types of fat raise blood cholesterol levels, and other types of fat cause a lowering of the blood cholesterol.

Dietary fats are classified in three types: *saturated*, *monounsaturated*, and *polyunsaturated*. The type of fat that raises the cholesterol level most dramatically is *saturated fats*. They are found in meat and high-fat dairy products, such as butter and whole milk. Saturated fats are easily recognized because they are always solid at room temperature. Examples of saturated fats are butter, vegetable shortening, and lard. *Polyunsaturated fats*, when substituted for saturated fats, will lower the cholesterol in the blood. *Monounsaturated fats* are found in foods such as peanuts and peanut oil, olives and olive oil, and avocados. Recent research information shows evidence that monounsaturated fats are at least as effective as polyunsaturates in lowering blood cholesterol. Both of these fats are commonly found in vegetable oils and remain liquid at room temperature.

FOODS HIGH IN SATURATED FATS

- Lard
- Butter
- Fatty cuts of beef, pork, and lamb
- Coconut oil
- Palm Oil

(Coconut oil and Palm Oil: Commonly used in commercially prepared cookies, pies, and non-dairy creamers)

- Cream
- Whole milk (4%)
- Hard cheeses made from cream

FOODS WITH HIDDEN FATS

- Marbled meats
- Creamed, fried, buttery, and au gratin prepared foods
- Hard cheese
- Deep-fried foods
- Cream soups
- Ice cream
- Chocolate
- Coffee creamer
- Granola (most)
- Pies, cakes, and cookies
- Processed meats, such as hot dogs and bologna
- Salad dressings

The overall fat content of your diet should be low (less than 30% of your daily intake of calories), and it should consist largely of unsaturated fats. To replace the fat calories in your diet, increase your consumption of carbohydrates and fiber, such as whole wheat bread and pasta, vegetables, fruits, grilled or baked fish, and skinless poultry.

Some fat is easy to see, such as fat on meat and fried foods. Much of the fat you eat is hidden. Examples of hidden fat foods include the following:

- 100% fat: Cooking oils, vegetable shortening, lard, mayonnaise, margarine, butter
- 75% fat: Cheese, nuts, peanut butter, salad dressings, luncheon meats, bologna, spam, hot dogs, bacon, sausage, and most steak
- 50% fat: Chocolate, chips, pies, pastries, ice cream, cookies

Remember that whether you are eating at home or away from home you should read food labels, eat smaller servings, and eat fewer fried foods. Fill up with vegetables or salads (with fat-free dressing), and most importantly, be aware of the nutritional content of what you are eating.

Understanding Food Labels: What Does "Fat Content" Mean?

Food labels report fat content in grams. If you eat 2000 calories each day, 30% or less of your daily diet should come from fat. In this example 30% of 2000 calories is 600 calories. Each gram of fat produces 9 calories. Therefore 600 calories divided by 9 calories/gram = 66 grams of fat. This should be the limit each day for a 2000 calorie diet.

TYPE AND PERCENTAGE OF FAT

TYPE OF OIL	Saturated	Polyunsaturated	Monounsaturated	Other Fats
Coconut Oil	77%	2%	6%	15%
Palm Oil	51%	10%	39%	0
Cotton Seed Oil	27%	54%	19%	0
Peanut Oil	13%	33%	49%	5%
Soybean Oil	15%	61%	24%	0
Olive Oil	14%	9%	77%	0
Corn Oil	13%	62%	25%	0
Sunflower Oil	11%	69%	20%	0
Safflower Oil	9%	78%	12%	1%
Canola Oil	6%	31%	62%	1%

Diet Guidelines for a Healthy Heart

These guidelines offer a brief summary of three diets for a healthy heart. If your doctor has prescribed one of these diets for you, you need more complete information. The American Heart Association has free pamphlets available that explain the low-cholesterol and low-sodium diets in detail.

Reading labels

Labels on packaged foods make it easier to select healthier products, but you must understand how to interpret them. If the product makes any nutritional claim, the label lists two categories of information. **"Nutritional Information per Serving"** lists the amount of calories, protein, carbohydrates, fat, and sodium (salt) in one serving. It also tells you how much is considered *one* serving, which can be confusing. For example, one normal serving of milk is 1 cup, or 8 ounces. If you pour milk into a tall drinking glass, however, you may have 10 to 16 ounces.

The second category is **"Percentage of U.S. Recommended Daily Allowances (U.S. RDA)"** for protein, vitamins, and minerals in each serving. Remember that these numbers are percentages, so if the label on a milk carton says "Protein 20," this means that 1 cup provides 20% of the protein you need each day.

Packaged foods that do not claim to provide nutrition do not have these labels, but they do list the ingredients. The largest quantity is listed first and the smallest amount last. For example, a jar of sweet pickles lists the ingredients as "Cucumbers, water, corn syrup, vinegar, peppers, salt, natural and artificial flavors, preservatives, and artificial coloring." This tells you cucumbers are the main ingredient, water the next highest ingredient, and so forth.

Of course, fresh meats, fish and seafood, fruits, and vegetables, do not carry labels. You need to learn which ones are the best for your diet and which ones to avoid.

Low-cholesterol diet

The average American consumes a large amount of cholesterol every day: men about 500 milligrams (mg) and women about 320 mg. A low-cholesterol diet limits cholesterol intake to less than 300 mg a day. To manage this, only 30% (or less) of the total calories you eat every day should come from fat. In addition, most of this fat should come from **polyunsaturated fat,** the "good" fat that helps lower blood cholesterol.

How can you tell the difference between "good" and "bad" fat? Polyunsaturated oil is usually liquid and comes from vegetables such as corn, cottonseed, soybean, sunflower, and safflower. Peanut, canola, and olive oil are **monounsaturated fats** that are neutral and do not add cholesterol. The "bad" fats are **saturated fats,** which harden at room temperature and are found in meat, dairy products made from whole milk or cream, solid and hydrogenated shortening, coconut oil, palm oil, and cocoa butter.

Here are some tips for avoiding too much saturated fat:

1. Eat less meat. Adults need about 5-7 ounces of meat, poultry, fish, or seafood a day.
2. Avoid "prime grade" or heavily marbled meats, corned beef, pastrami, regular ground beef, frankfurters, sausage, bacon, lunch meat, goose, duck, or organ meats. Select very lean cuts of meat. Trim skin off chicken and turkey.
3. Avoid fried meat, chicken, fish, or seafood. Use a rack to drain off fat when broiling, baking, or roasting.
4. Eat no more than two whole eggs (yolks and whites) per week. (Egg whites are allowed, since they contain little cholesterol.)
5. Avoid dairy products containing more than 1% milk fat, such as butter, sour cream, cream cheese, creamed cottage cheese, and most natural and processed cheeses. Select milk products that contain only up to 1% milk fat. Use polyunsaturated margarine.
6. Avoid packaged foods or bakery items that contain egg yolks, whole milk, saturated fats, cream sauces, or butter. Select only those that have a low-cholesterol rating.
7. Avoid cashews, coconut, pistachios, and macadamia nuts. Most other types of vegetables, fruits, nuts, and seeds are low in cholesterol.

Low-sodium diet

The average American consumes about 1 to 2 teaspoons of salt every day, 6 to 18 grams, and most of this salt is added at the table. Your body needs only about 0.5 grams of salt a day. Since most foods that come from animals (meat, poultry, fish, eggs, milk) are naturally high in sodium, your body's requirements are easily met without adding salt to your food.

What is the difference between salt and sodium? Sodium keeps the right amount of water in your body, so some is necessary for good health. However, too much sodium causes water retention, which raises your blood pressure.

It may take a little time to get used to a low-sodium diet, particularly if you are accustomed to eating highly salted foods. Start by eliminating salt from the table. Use spices and herbs that contain no sodium to add flavor, and try some of the new salt substitutes that contain no sodium.

Many packaged and processed foods are now marketed as low sodium, including cheeses, luncheon meats, canned and packaged food, and even snacks such as potato chips. However, beware if the package reads "reduced sodium"; the sodium content may still be too high. If you are not sure of a product, read the ingredients carefully and look for the words "salt, sodium, soda, baking powder, monosodium glutamate (MSG), and disodium phosphate." If you are still in doubt, do not eat it.

Here are some tips for eliminating the "hidden" sodium from your diet:

1. Avoid cured or smoked meat, poultry, or fish. These include ham, bacon, corned beef, regular luncheon meats, sausage, commercially frozen fish, canned fish packed in oil or brine, and canned shellfish.
2. Avoid frozen, canned, and dehydrated main-dish foods such as pizza, TV dinners, spaghetti, chili, stews, and soups.
3. Avoid canned vegetables and vegetable juices.
4. Avoid cheese, buttermilk, and cocoa mixes.
5. Avoid commercial sauces (catsup, chili sauce, steak sauce, soy sauce), mayonnaise, salad dressing, olives, pickles, meat tenderizers, and seasoning salts.

Low-calorie diet

Losing weight (or keeping weight off) is an important part of controlling blood pressure and reducing blood cholesterol levels. Your doctor, a dietitian, or a nutritionist can advise you about calories, since this depends on how active you are, your height, and your physical condition.

The low-cholesterol diet is an excellent basis for a weight loss program. Fats are high in calories, and the low-cholesterol diet is essentially a low-fat diet. For example, 1 cup of whole milk contains 150 calories, but the same amount of skim milk has only 86 calories. Also, because it emphasizes fresh fruits and vegetables and discourages processed foods, the low-cholesterol diet is nutritionally well balanced.

Weight loss should be gradual. Remember: it probably took you several years to put the pounds on, so expect it to take several months to lose them.

Here are some other tips for helping you lose weight:

1. Divide your daily calorie allowance into several small meals a day, instead of eating one or two large meals.
2. For between-meal snacks, choose high-fiber, low-calorie foods such as apples or celery. High-fiber foods make your stomach feel full quicker.
3. For between-meal hunger pangs, fool your stomach with a glass of ice water, hot tea, or calorie-free soda.
4. If you eat when you're bored, busy yourself to take your mind off food. Change your activity—do something you enjoy, take a walk, or take a shower.
5. If you eat when you are "blue," try the "buddy system" with a dieting friend. Agree to call each other for help whenever you're tempted to indulge.
6. Regular exercise that burns calories (walking, jogging, swimming, etc.) is the magic ingredient in many people's exercise programs. Check with your doctor first about the safest program for you.
7. "Too good to be true" weight loss programs are just that—they are either worthless or dangerous. Follow a diet that has been medically recommended and skip the "fad" diets.

Nutrition and Diet for Older Adults

As you become older, a well-balanced diet is very important. Many times, because of such factors as decreased activity, life stresses, chewing difficulties, and decreased appetite, older adults do not maintain an optimal diet for their age and body build. The following guidelines help to promote your health and prevent disease.

General Food Requirements

Daily nourishment should consist of the foods in the food pyramid:

Fiber: Fiber is an important component of a well-balanced diet. It absorbs water, which adds bulk to the food passing through the gastrointestinal tract. This is turn helps to prevent constipation. Fiber also helps to prevent diverticular disease and cancer of the large intestine.

Foods High in Fiber

- Unrefined cereals
- Fruit
- Vegetables
- Legumes

Calories: It is well known that older adults who are significantly underweight or overweight are less healthy than those who are close to the average weight for their sex, height, and build.

It is commonly reported that older men require between 1200 and 1500 calories per day and women require between 1000 and 1300 calories per day to maintain their body energy balance and vital functioning. As an older adult, you require nutrtional foods that are high in minerals and vitamins, but which are not high in calories. Because it is often difficult to get the needed vitamins and minerals without eating at least 1200 calories a day, it is important for you to exercise to burn the excess calories.

Food Guide Pyramid
A Guide to Daily Food Choices

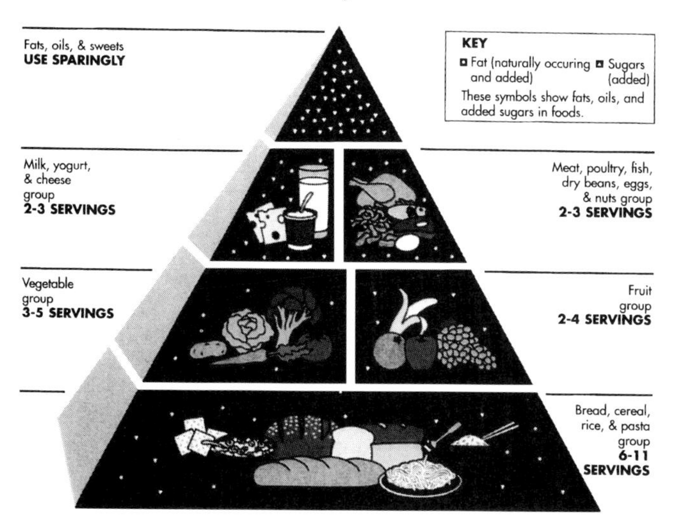

Calcium: Both men and women may experience age-related bone loss. This may result in osteoporosis. To ensure that they are getting adequate calcium, post-menopausal women and older men should have between 1000 and 1500 milligrams of calcium every day, either through diet or by taking a diet supplement.

Calcium Sources

- 8 ounces of milk (roughly 300 mg of calcium)
- Low-fat yogurt
- Non-fat dry milk
- Fish and shell fish such as oysters, shrimp, canned sardines
- Dark green vegetables such as collard, turnip, mustard greens, kale, and broccoli
- Calcium supplements such as calcium tablets or powders (consult your health care provider to determine the type and amount to take)

Iron, Vitamin B^{12}, and Folic Acid: Anemia and vitamin deficiencies are not a normal consequence of aging. Poor diet, alcohol, or diseases such as iron deficiency anemia, vitamin B^{12} deficiency, and folic acid deficiency may cause anemia. In addition, medications such as aspirin or nonsteroidal antiinflammatory drugs (Motrin, Nalfon, Pontstel, and Naprosyn) may cause irritation to the stomach lining and the intestines, which may cause chronic blood loss in the stool. If your health care provider recommends that you need more iron, you may either take an iron supplement or you may make sure that your diet is rich in iron.

Sources of Iron, B^{12}, and Folic Acid

IRON
- Liver or lean red meat
- Whole grain or enriched breads and cereals
- Rice and pasta (enriched)
- Nuts
- Broccoli, spinach, and kale

FOLIC ACID
- Fresh, green, leafy vegetables
- Mushrooms
- Liver
- Lima and kidney beans
- Whole grain bread
- Nuts

VITAMIN B^{12} **(all animal products)**
- Liver, pork, beef, and lamb
- Poultry
- Fish
- Eggs
- Low-fat milk
- Oysters

Sodium: Studies now show that most Americans, including the older population, consume more dietary salt than the body requires. This may result in the body retaining fluid, and may play a vital role in high blood-pressure. As a rule, fresh, frozen, and canned fruits and fruit juices are low in sodium, as are fresh or frozen vegetables and grain products cooked without salt. Milk and dairy products, and meat, poultry, and fish contain varying amounts of salt. It is very important to read package labels to determine the sodium content of boxed and prepared foods.

What is Osteoporosis?

Osteoporosis is the most common metabolic bone disease. It results from the loss of calcium in the bones, causing the bones to become brittle and susceptible to breaking. Osteoporosis, which means "porous bone," is also called the "silent disease," because it is usually not diagnosed until the person suffers a fracture, or broken bone. Osteoporosis affects 15 million to 20 million people in the United States. Women are affected eight times more often than men.

Osteoporosis primarily affects the vertebrae and the hips, wrists, and rib bones. Fractures can occur without any outside force being placed on the bones, especially in the spinal column. Hip bones are most often broken. Women suffer hip fractures two to three times more often than men. The vertebrae may compress and cause a stooped appearance or outward curvature of the back. The result is loss of height and back pain.

How do bones function?

Bone is a living tissue that is being formed and shaped continuously. Bones go through a process of formation (building up the bone) and resorption (breaking down the bone for other uses) throughout your life. Bones store calcium for other body functions, and the body takes the calcium out by resorption. Bone mass, or the amount of bone in your body, increases as you grow through childhood, adolescence, and into adulthood. Bone mass is at its greatest when you are about 35 years of age. Up to that time the process of formation occurs faster than the process of resorption. However, as you age, resorption naturally occurs faster than formation, resulting in a gradual decrease in bone mass. Bones become brittle and susceptible to fractures. Women suffer the greatest loss of bone mass within the first 5 years after menopause (the ceasing of menstruation). The decrease in bone mass is slower in men.

Why are women affected more often?

One out of four women, and half the women over 65 years of age, have osteoporosis to some extent. Most are white women who have gone through menopause. Generally, blacks have greater bone mass than whites, and men have greater bone mass than women. Petite women with small bones and thin bodies have very small bone masses. Thus women are at greater risk of developing osteoporosis if they are white, Asian, or are petite.

Osteoporosis is also caused by low estrogen levels that occur in women after menopause. Although the role of estrogen is not clear, it is linked to the processes of bone formation and resorption. Estrogen is thought to reduce bone resorption, to reduce calcium loss through the kidneys, and to increase calcium absorption in the digestive tract. Estrogen protects women who have had an inadequate intake of calcium in their growing years. However, when estrogen levels drop after menopause, bone resorption in women increases greatly.

What are the risk factors?

Two major factors for osteoporosis are lack of exercise and inadequate intake of calcium, vitamin D, and protein. Osteoporosis caused by calcium and vitamin D deficiencies affects men and women 70 to 85 years of age. Other risk factors contributing to the disease are these:

1. A family history of osteoporosis
2. Smoking and consuming too much alcohol and caffeine, which interfere with the absorption of calcium
3. Prolonged use of drugs or medications such as steroids, magnesium-based antacids such as Maalox, and heparin
4. Diseases and hormonal disorders such as rheumatoid arthritis, liver disease, certain cancers, and an overactive thyroid
5. Poor calcium absorption in the intestines

Although osteoporosis primarily affects middle-aged or older people, it can occur in young adults. Injuries that result in paralysis or long periods of immobility can lead to osteoporosis.

How is osteoporosis diagnosed?

Osteoporosis is diagnosed by several methods. A physical examination can reveal bone thinning. X-rays can show bone loss of 25% to 40% or more, but they are only helpful in later detection. A more specialized x-ray technique (computed tomography) can detect bone loss as slight as 2%, which is useful in measuring a patient's response to therapy. Absorptiometry, another specialized x-ray technique, can detect bone loss of as little as 2% in the wrist and hand.

Therapeutic Exercise: Focus on Walking

What exactly is meant by "therapeutic exercise"?

Therapeutic exercise is the motion of the body or its parts to achieve symptom-free movement and function. It is used to develop and retrain deficient muscles; to restore as much normal movement as possible to prevent deformity; to stimulate the functions of various organs and body systems; to build strength and endurance; and to promote relaxation.

Various theories and methods have been proposed to improve health through exercise and movement. Decreased physical activity, which may be the result of illness or treatment, can lead to anxiety, depression, weakness, fatigue, and nausea. Regular, moderate exercise can prevent these feelings and help a person feel energetic.

Aerobic exercise (the sustained rhythmic activity of large muscle groups, which entails using large amounts of oxygen) increases heart rate, stroke volume, respiratory rate, and relaxation of blood vessels. Cardiovascular fitness and increased stamina are the goals. Body fat is also reduced. Aerobic exercises include running, jogging, brisk walking, swimming, aquadynamics, and aerobic dance.

Always check with your doctor before beginning any exercise program and for help in choosing the type of exercise program that is best for you. Whatever type you choose, the goal should be to maintain a regular, moderate exercise program to enhance physical and emotional health. The exercise should involve large muscle groups in dynamic movement for about 20 minutes 3 or more days a week. The exertion should be within limits appropriate to your physical status and needs. At the end of exercise you should feel replenished rather than bored, burned out, or excessively fatigued.

What makes walking a good form of regular exercise?

Walking allows for psychomotor expression without the hazards of contact sports and is adaptable to a wide range of weather or geographic conditions, schedules, personalities, and body types. It can be social or asocial, organized or unorganized as an activity. The long-term effects on joints and organs of regular, sustained, vigorous walking currently are unknown; physicians do report a lower incidence of the type of musculoskeletal damage resulting from the "pounding" effects of jogging.

Making time for exercising regularly is hard. What can I do to make it easier?

There are two major obstacles to overcome in undertaking and maintaining an exercise program: making exercise part of a life-style and avoiding injury. Suggestions for making exercise a safe part of a life-style include:

1. Start in small increments, and keep it fun.
2. Avoid exercising for 2 hours after a large meal, and do not eat for 1 hour after exercising.
3. Include at least 10 minutes of warm-up and cool-down exercises.
4. Use proper equipment and clothing.
5. Post goals, pictures of the ideal self, and notes of encouragement in a readily seen place for self-encouragement.
6. Use visualization daily to picture successful attainment of exercise benefit (for example, looking toned or graceful or achieving an ideal weight).
7. Keep records of weekly measures of weight, blood pressure, and pulse.
8. Focus on the rewards of exercise; keep a record of feelings, and compare differences in relaxation, energy, concentration, and sleep patterns.
9. Work with a peer or join a structured exercise class, running club, or fitness center. Spend more time with people dedicated to wellness.
10. Stop exercising or at least slow down and consult with a practitioner if any unusual, unexplainable symptoms occur.
11. Reward yourself for working toward exercise goals as well as attaining them. For example, after a month in an exercise program, buy a new pair of running shoes or treat yourself to a special wish.

What does a walking (or "rhythmic walking") program entail?

Rhythmic walking consists of walking briskly, arms swinging, so your whole body is involved in the rhythm of your movement and your heart rate is increased. It is a regular program to benefit every system of your body.

A good exercise plan starts slowly, allowing your body time to adjust. It is important that you do something to exercise the whole body on a regular basis. *Regular* means every day, or at least every other day; build up to about 20 minutes 3 or more days a week. The right kind of exercise never makes you feel sore, stiff, or exhausted.

We repeat: *first check with your doctor.* Before starting a program, it is important to know if there are precautions you need to take. This is especially important if you have high blood pressure, diabetes, joint or bone problems, or heart disease. People with these conditions can exercise, but they must follow certain guidelines to do it safely.

Rhythmic walking is inexpensive. It requires no special equipment or uniforms. Wear comfortable clothes in which you can move freely. You must have the right kind of shoes. Running or jogging shoes or the shoes specially designed for walking are good. The wrong shoes can cause painful damage, such as tendonitis. Select shoes designed for walking, jogging, or running; look for a shock-absorbent cushioning midsole. A watch with a second hand to measure your heart rate is also important.

Everyone who exercises outside the home should carry identification and change for a telephone call and money for a taxi. Some people like to carry a small water bottle such as a plastic soda bottle. To carry these items, a small backpack or hip pack leaves your hands free to swing.

If it is wet, slippery, or hot, or if you feel unsafe walking in your neighborhood, enclosed shopping malls can be great places for walking. Some malls open early, before the shopping crowds arrive, especially for people who want to walk.

How hard should I exercise?

Your heart rate is the best indicator of how hard your body is working. As you work harder, your heart rate increases; as you slow down, your heart rate decreases. You can take your pulse to measure your heart rate. To experience the benefits of exercise, you need to work hard enough to get your heart rate up to a certain point, called the *training heart rate,* and keep it there. Your nurse or doctor can tell you what your training heart rate should be and how to take your own pulse. Find these two things out before beginning your exercise regimen.

How long should I exercise?

It is important to start exercising slowly and build up gradually. If you have been very ill or have not been exercising on a regular basis, start with a 5- or 10-minute walk and add 2 minutes each week. If you are able to build up endurance without problems, work up to 45 minutes daily or every other day. More than 60 minutes of rhythmic walking daily is not necessary.

A good work-out consists of three phases: warm-up, training period, and cool-down. The warm-up is necessary to prepare the body for exercise. Warm up by walking slowly. Next, begin rhythmic walking. This is your training period. Work up to your target heart rate, and walk steadily for your set period of time. Finally, walk slowly to cool off. The cool-down is necessary to help your body recover and to prevent soreness or stiffness.

If you are exercising correctly, you should never feel exhausted after the cool-down. If you do, slow down and take it easier next time. If you feel fatigued for hours after exercise or if you feel sore and stiff, you have done too much or exercised incorrectly.

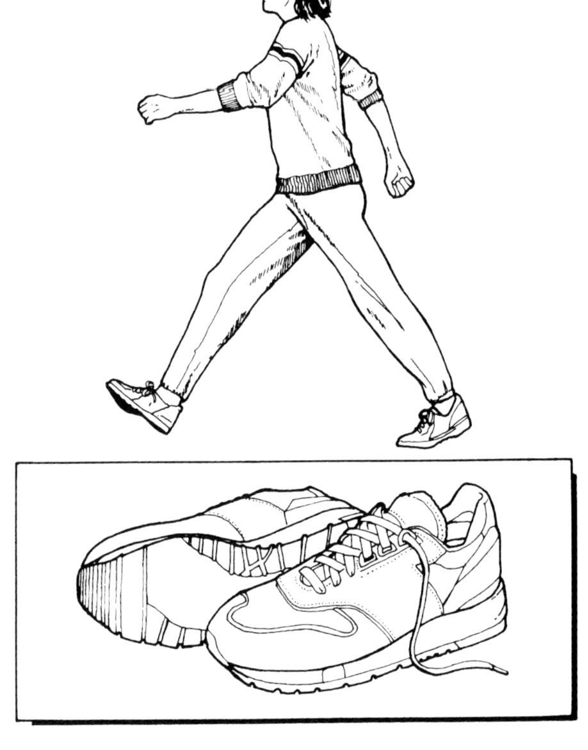

Home Safety and Fall Prevention

Unintentional injury is the third leading cause of death and disability for persons over 65 years of age. The disability that may result from an injury may end the independence of an older person living at home. Falls are the leading cause of injury for the older adult. Because the bones in the body may become more brittle with aging, a fall may potentially cause a serious injury. A hip fracture secondary to a fall may be a catastrophic event for an older person. Most falls in the older adult occur because of an environmental hazard, loss of muscle strength and coordination, an impaired sense of balance, and slowing reaction time. To ensure the safety of an older person, and to help prevent falls and other injuries, it is important to make the person's living space safe and free from hazards.

Environmental Safety

- Steps should be highly visible, have good lighting, nonskid treads, and handrails.
- A strong banister running along all indoor and outdoor steps is essential.
- Clearly mark and light the top and bottom steps.
- Use bright lighting in the living space.
- Remove all floor clutter in the walkways.
- Remove slippery floor coverings such as polished linoleum, small mats, and area or throw rugs.
- Use nonskid floor wax, wall-to-wall carpeting, or rubber-backed rugs. Tack down the corners of area rugs.
- Install nonskid mats and handrails in the bathtub and near the toilet and bed.
- A bedside lamp or low-wattage night-light should be available in the bedroom.
- Secure electrical cords along the walls or baseboards.
- Store frequently used dishes, clothes, and other items within easy reach; climbing on a stool or chair should be avoided.
- Set the temperature on the hot water heater to no hotter than 130° F or have a mixing valve installed on the bathtub faucet to prevent burns.

Personal Safety Activities

- If you need glasses, wear them, but never walk around with glasses that are meant only for reading. Take them off before moving around.
- If you are even slightly unsteady on your feet, use a cane. Do not hesitate to use a walker either inside the house or outdoors.
- Always turn lights on and use adequate wattage light bulbs to brighten the room.
- Wear wide-base, low-heel shoes with corrugated soles to help prevent slips and falls.
- Do not wear flimsy or slippery-soled shoes or slippers.
- When getting up at night, first sit on the edge of the bed to make sure you are awake and steady, then turn on a light before walking to the bathroom or around the room.
- Don't ever smoke in bed. If you are sleepy, don't light up a cigarette regardless of where you are sitting.
- Always wear clothing with short sleeves when you are cooking. Never reach over a hot burner on the stove.
- If you live alone, have a safety plan to call for help or to get assistance.
- If you take a medication that makes you dizzy or weak, discuss these symptoms with your health care provider. Being dizzy or weak when you get up to walk or go down stairs may increase your risk of falling.

Exercise and Activity for Older Adults

Exercise is believed to influence both the length and quality of life. Most research findings clearly show that exercise improves both overall physical capacity and heart function in the older adult, especially when done often enough and long enough. Experts agree that it is possible for healthy older adults to delay the physiologic changes in the body by exercising daily.

Another important benefit of exercise is its ability to help with weight control. The problem of overweight may be caused as much by inactivity as by overeating. For example, an excess of only 100 calories a day can produce a 10-pound weight gain in 1 year; on the other hand, those extra calories can be burned up during a 15- to 20-minute daily walk.

BENEFITS OF EXERCISE

- Improves circulation and heart function
- Improves oxygen uptake from the blood
- Improves lung function
- Improves the body's use of glucose
- Assists with weight control
- Strengthens bones
- Helps to decrease general aches and pains
- Improves mobility of the joints
- Improves outlook by feeling and looking well
- Strengthens muscles
- Builds endurance
- Improves posture

Establish an Exercise Program

Before beginning a new exercise program, it is important to meet with your regular health care provider to ensure that the exercise program you are planning is appropriate for your current physical health. Regardless of the type of exercise program you choose, it should meet three criteria: (1) the exercise should agree with your physical ability; (2) it should make sufficient demands on the body to be beneficial; and (3) most important, it should be enjoyable.

EXERCISE POINTERS

- Record your heart rate (pulse) before you begin to exercise and again during your exercise.
- Start gradually—especially if you have been inactive.
- Increase the amount of exercise daily.
- Breathe deeply and evenly when you exercise.
- Rest whenever you need to during exercise.
- Exercise with friends or play lively music when you exercise.
- Rest for a few minutes before continuing if you become short of breath or dizzy.
- Write on the calendar or in a notebook the date when you started to exercise. Each time you exercise, record the time and how you felt when you finished.

Exercise comes in many forms, from skiing to water aerobics. What type of exercise you choose to do is not as important as choosing the best exercise for you—one that you will find enjoyable and that you will keep doing. Two of the most common types of exercise are walking and aerobics.

Walking: Walking does much more than just tone and strengthen the muscles. It also eases the mind, and is relaxing and energizing. Walking is not a new exercise, for long ago Hippocrates recognized walking as beneficial and called it "man's best medicine." Compared with other exercises, walking is relatively injury- and stress-free on the body.

45-MINUTE EXERCISES

Exercise	Calories Used
Brisk fitness walk up hill (10 degree incline)	540 calories
Jogging	455 calories
Moderate fitness walk up hill (5 degree incline)	338 calories
Tennis (singles)	311 calories
Fitness walk (4 mph)	248 calories
Bicycling (5.5 mph)	203 calories
Dancing	162 calories
Slow walking (2 mph)	113 calories

Source: Walking, January 1986, page 18.

Aerobics: Aerobic exercises include such things as fast walking, running, swimming, and bicycling. They should be done continuously for a sustained period of time without starting and stopping. During this time, the supply of oxygen to the muscle is adequate for their needs. The object of the exercises is to improve the body's efficiency in processing oxygen for use by the body's organs, such as the heart and the lungs. Although aerobic activity is more strenuous than walking, the benefits from the exercise are significant.

Weight Training: Just because you are older does not mean that you cannot choose an activity such as weight training. If you think that you might like to weight train, discuss the idea with your health care provider and obtain medical clearance before beginning the training. Weight training stresses the entire skeletal system and thus helps to decrease bone loss. It also builds upper body strength and improves overall fitness.

It does not matter what type of exercise you choose. The important thing is to choose an exercise that you have the capability to do and will enjoy doing. Then commit yourself to the exercise and do it routinely, at least 20 minutes three or more times each week. Your mind and body will thank you.

Preventing Respiratory Infections

Respiratory infections can be a serious complication for anyone with a chronic lung disease. Unfortunately, people with chronic lung diseases are more susceptible to respiratory infections; even an ordinary cold that causes only sniffles in someone else can turn into pneumonia. Because of this, you must make every effort to prevent infection. You must also learn the early danger signs and see your doctor at once when any symptoms appear.

Preventing Infection

Follow your doctor's orders. Take your medications exactly as ordered. Perform chest physiotherapy as directed. If oxygen therapy is prescribed, take it as ordered.

Take care of yourself every day. Drink at least six glasses of water daily (unless your doctor tells you differently). Eat a nutritious, well-balanced diet. Sleep 7 or 8 hours every night. Take several short rests during the day. Learn to conserve your energy and avoid getting too tired.

Stay away from people who have colds and flu, if at all possible. If this cannot be avoided, wear a disposable mask (available at medical supply companies and many grocery stores) when around people with colds or flu.

Avoid air pollution, including tobacco smoke, wood or oil smoke, car exhaust, and industrial pollution.

Take special precautions with your personal hygiene. Wash your hands before taking your medication or handling your oxygen equipment. Wash your hands after handling soiled tissues and before and after using the bathroom. Always rinse your oral inhaler after each use.

Ask your doctor about flu vaccines.

Detecting infections

Symptoms of respiratory infections can appear suddenly and worsen quickly. When an infection develops, it is important to start treatment right away. Your doctor may decide to prescribe antibiotics or other drugs to get the infection under control before it becomes serious. (**Do not try to treat yourself.** Over-the-counter cold remedies may worsen the problem, so do not use them unless your doctor tells you it is okay.) Call your doctor immediately if any of these signs occur:

- Fever
- Increased coughing, wheezing, or trouble breathing
- Mucus changes in any of these ways: the mucus is thicker; the amount is either more or less than usual; it has a foul odor; or the color is green, yellow, brown, pink, or red
- Stuffy nose, sneezing, or sore throat
- Increased fatigue or weakness
- Weight gain or loss of more than 5 pounds within a week
- Swollen ankles or feet
- Confusion, memory loss, or persistent drowsiness

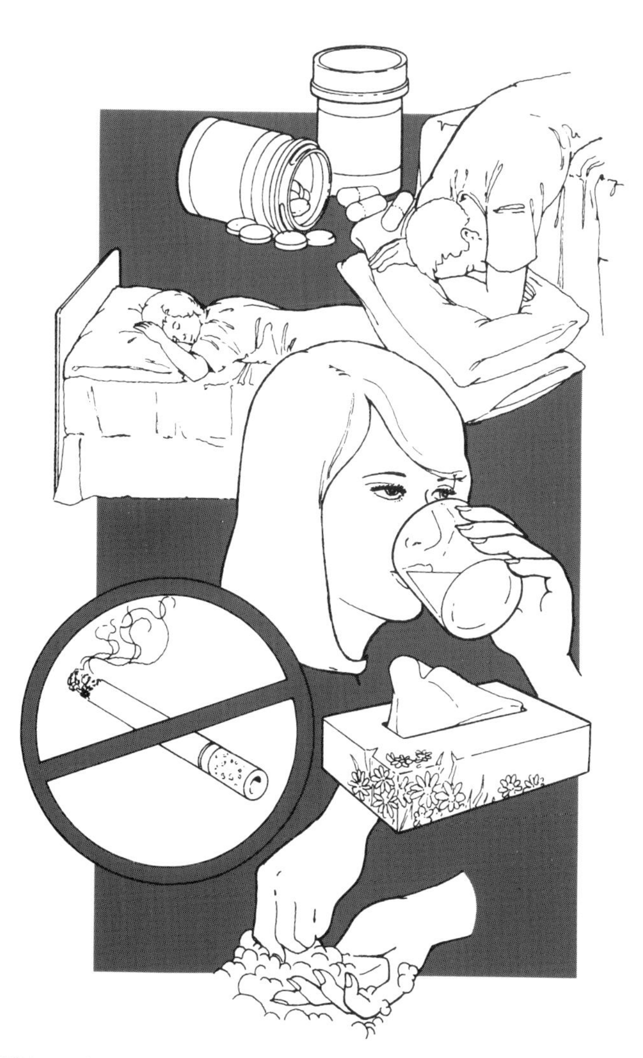

Smoking and Your Lungs

Chances are, you started smoking because it was cool, sophisticated, and glamorous. Or your friends smoked and you were curious about what smoking was like.

Now you know smoking is anything but cool. It makes you cough, cuts your "wind," gives you bad breath, and stains your teeth. It's also expensive; in one year, a heavy smoker may spend $1,000 or more on cigarettes.

More important, smoking causes emphysema, chronic bronchitis, lung cancer, heart disease, and gum disease. It increases your chances of having a stroke, diseases of the blood vessels, and stomach ulcers. Women who smoke during pregnancy may have premature babies. Smoking increases the risk of osteoporosis in women. And smoke in the air harms nonsmokers.

You and your defense system

The insides of your lungs are exposed to the environment every time you breathe. To protect them from foreign particles that could enter the body through this route, the lungs have several defense mechanisms.

Tiny hairlike cilia line your bronchial tubes. Normally they are in constant movement, sweeping germs, dirt, and mucus out of your lungs. But tobacco smoke slows down and actually paralyzes the cilia. Dirt particles and germs that enter the lungs are not removed. And the mucus that collects in the lungs provides a fertile environment for germs to multiply. This is the reason smokers suffer more respiratory infections.

Mucus lining the airways serves two purposes: it helps remove dirt and germs and it moistens the air you breathe. Smoking dries out the mucus, further hampering the defensive action of removing foreign matter. Smokers often experience dry, scratchy throat because the normal moisture is absent.

The chemicals in tobacco

Tar is a cancer-causing substance that clings to the inside of your lungs, forming a brown, sticky coat. All tobacco contains tar. Many people switch to low-tar cigarettes in the belief that these brands were less damaging. But the fact is, even small amounts of tar can still cause cancer. In addition, many smokers who switch to low-tar brands take deeper draws and smoke more cigarettes.

Nicotine causes the blood vessels to constrict, raising your blood pressure and forcing your heart to work harder than it should. Smokers suffer from cold hands and feet caused by poor circulation. In time, this can cause vascular diseases.

Burning tobacco produces carbon monoxide. Each time you inhale the hot smoke, you are taking carbon monoxide into your lungs. The tiny blood vessels in your lungs pick up this carbon monoxide instead of oxygen. Tests on smokers have found that carbon monoxide levels in their blood are 15 times higher than in the blood of nonsmokers. As a smoker, your entire body is chronically oxygen-deficient.

It's not too late to quit

Even if you have been smoking for years—even if you already have a lung disease—quitting smoking now will greatly improve your health. The cilia will begin working again and help keep your lungs swept clean. Your blood vessels will relax, allowing the blood to flow normally, so your heart will no longer work so hard. Your lung tissue will become healthier and you will breathe easier.

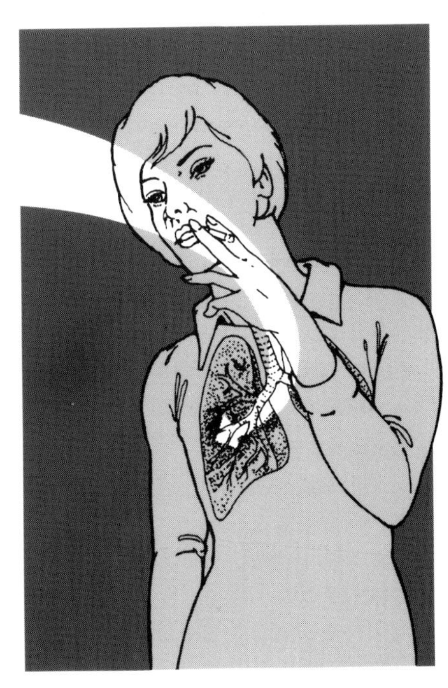

Quitting Smoking

Your doctor has told you to quit smoking. You want to, but you aren't sure of the best way. Perhaps you've tried before. Or you're afraid you'll gain weight.

What's the best way to quit?

There are many ways to quit smoking, but you need only one thing—*the desire to quit*. Once you have that all-important ingredient, you will succeed.

You can quit "cold turkey," or you can set a quit date and taper off gradually over a 2-week period. Some people find it helpful to have support from others who are quitting at the same time. Your local chapter of the American Lung Association, the American Cancer Society, or the American Heart Association, or a hospital in your community can help you locate a smoking cessation class. Or, you can use the "buddy system"—make a pact with a friend who wants to quit and provide support for each other.

Many people find chewing nicotine gum or using a nicotine patch helpful for the first few weeks. Talk to your doctor about prescribing one of these for you.

Adopt as many techniques as you think will work for you, and use them all.

What about withdrawal symptoms?

Keep in mind that most smokers actually have a double addiction: physical and psychological. You will need to deal with both aspects.

Physical withdrawal can be a problem for heavy smokers (more than one pack a day). The symptoms vary from one person to another, but common complaints are headaches, constipation, irritability, nervousness, trouble concentrating, and insomnia. You may even cough more for the first week after quitting as your cilia became active again. This is actually a sign that your body is healing itself.

You can do several things to ease the withdrawal symptoms. Although you may fear that you'll be craving a cigarette all the time, each urge actually lasts only 2 or 3 minutes. When it hits, do a minute or two of deep-breathing exercises to calm the urge; close your eyes, take a deep breath, and slowly let it out. If you still feel a craving, change your activity—walk around or do something that requires both hands, or do something that you especially enjoy.

Drink lots of water to help flush the toxins from your body. Eat a healthy, well-balanced diet. Many authorities say that eating less meat and more fresh vegetables and fruits helps reduce withdrawal symptoms. To combat aftermeal cravings, leave the table immediately and brush your teeth. Sugarless gum or hard candy, a toothpick, or unsalted, shelled sunflower seeds satisfy the oral craving without adding calories.

Daily exercise (unless your doctor advises you not to) will help relax you and hasten recovery from the effects of nicotine.

Try to avoid situations that you associate with smoking, such as a morning cup of coffee or a before-dinner drink. You may need to modify your habits for a while until the withdrawal period is over. This also means avoiding spending much time around other smokers.

Write down all your reasons for quitting smoking to remind yourself whenever you're discouraged or tempted to smoke. Keep the list handy, and look at it often. And feel proud of yourself for quitting.

Won't I gain weight?

According to recent studies, only about one-third of ex-smokers gain some weight; one-third lose weight, and one-third stay the same. The key to not gaining weight is not to eat every time you crave a smoke. As long as you maintain a well-balanced diet, don't snack between meals, and exercise, you shouldn't experience any weight problems.

What if I fail?

Many people who have successfully quit smoking failed the first time they tried. Often they describe these "failures" as valuable learning experiences that helped them succeed the next time. Whatever you do, don't give up. More than 36 million American have already quit. You can, too.

Breathing Exercises

The feeling of not being able to get enough air into your lungs is frightening. Shortness of breath or difficulty breathing—called dyspnea—is a problem for people with chronic lung diseases. However, there are several things you can do to help you breathe more easily.

Avoiding trouble

Breathing pollutants can aggravate dyspnea. Avoid heavy traffic and smog as much as possible. Do not use aerosol sprays. Stay away from products that produce fumes, such as paint, kerosene, and cleaning agents.

Cold weather can trigger dyspnea. If you must go outside when it is cold, cover your mouth with a scarf or mask.

Very dry air increases dyspnea and thickens the mucus in your lungs. A portable room humidifier is helpful, especially in the winter.

Physical exertion brings on dyspnea. Learn to conserve your energy by resting frequently, alternating light and heavy tasks, and minimizing movement. Instead of standing, sit. Instead of pushing or lifting objects, pull. Be creative in managing tasks—for example, a cart or child's wagon can be used to haul groceries, and wheels can be installed on furniture that is frequently moved.

Breathing exercises

There are two simple exercises that can help you breathe more easily. You can do pursed lip breathing anywhere. With abdominal breathing, you will need to lie down. Practice them daily so that when you are having problems with dyspnea, you will immediately know what to do.

Pursed lip breathing

Pursed lip breathing will help get rid of the stale air trapped inside the lungs. It will slow down your breathing so that it is more efficient. (Breathing fast only makes the dyspnea worse.)

1. Breathe in slowly through your nose. Hold your breath for three seconds (count to yourself by saying one 100, two 100, three 100). Be sure to breathe through your nose to avoid gulping air.
2. Purse your lips as if you were going to whistle or give someone a kiss.
3. Breathe out slowly through your pursed lips for six seconds (count one 100, two 100, three 100, four 100, five 100, six 100.) The sound you make breathing out will be like a soft whistle.

Abdominal breathing

Abdominal breathing will also slow down your breathing to make it more effective. It also helps relax your entire body and is a wonderful technique to use before you go to sleep.

1. Lie on your back in a comfortable position with a pillow under head. Place another pillow under your knees to help relax your abdomen.
2. Rest one hand on your abdomen just below your rib cage. Rest the other hand on your chest.
3. Slowly breathe in and out through your nose using your abdominal muscles. The hand resting on your abdomen will rise when you breathe in, and it will fall when you breathe out. The hand on your chest should be almost still.

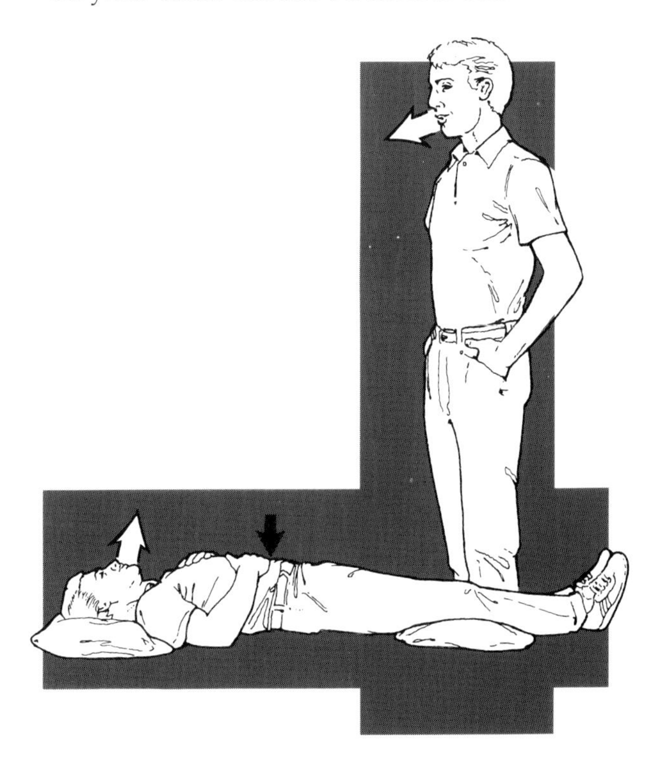

How to Use Ear Wash and Drops

You have been given a prescription that you should have filled at your own drugstore. You will also need a 2- or 3-ounce ear syringe, which you can buy at a drugstore if you do not have one.

Someone else should wash your ear for you

You cannot do it as well yourself. The instructions below should be followed very carefully:

1. Wash hands before and after this procedure.
2. Fill the ear syringe with the solution.
3. The solution must be at body temperature. If the solution is too warm or too cool, you will feel dizzy. Warm the solution by placing the syringe in a pan of hot water. Do *not* warm the solution on the stove.
4. Lie down with the ear to be washed facing up and pull up and out on the external ear. Place the tip of the ear syringe into the ear canal. Do not be afraid to push it down into the ear. However, you should get a return flow. If you do not, you have it in too far. Pull the syringe out slightly.
5. Pump the warmed solution from the syringe back and forth into the ear by squeezing and releasing the bulb of the syringe. Do this very vigorously and repeatedly. The ear wash must be forced back and forth, in and out of the ear canal.
6. Lean over and let the solution run out of the ear.
7. Pull the ear up, back, and out to straighten the ear canal.
8. Put three to five warmed drops into the ear.
9. If the solution burns too much at first, you may dilute the solution. Mix two ounces of water with two ounces of the solution. Later, decrease the amount of water used with each irrigation.
10. Use the solution and and drops twice a day for 2 weeks and then until the ear stops running or becomes dry. If you are not sure that the ear is dry, check it by putting a cotton swab down into the ear canal. If the cotton swab comes out dry, stop using the solution and drops. If the cotton swab is wet or there is an odor, continue using the solution and drops for 4 days.
11. Do not use the solution and drops as long as the ear remains dry and is not running, and as long as there is no odor. Should the ear start to run after being dry for a period of time, start using the ear solution and drops until the ear is dry again.
12. **Do not get any water in your ears.** You should not go swimming until you are told you may do so. Whenever there is a chance of getting water in your ears, such as when you shower or wash your hair, use cotton in the ear. First, place a dry piece of cotton in the ear and then a second piece that has been saturated with petroleum jelly.
13. If you have any questions, call your doctor.

Protecting Your Ears From Noise

Loud noises, or noise over a long period of time, can cause a permanent hearing loss. Noises also cause a temporary hearing loss, but over the years a permanent high-tone hearing loss develops. Protecting your ears from noise is necessary to keep normal hearing.

The best way to protect your ears is to avoid loud noise. Most of us don't have a choice; but if you are around loud noise, pay attention to your hearing. One way to monitor the presence of a hearing loss from noise is to listen for a ringing in your ears. If your ears ring, there is ear damage and possibly a hearing loss. A hearing loss from noise is permanent.

Any ear protection (also called noise defenders) is better than none at all. The best noise defender is one that is comfortable to wear. Different noise defenders are available, made from various materials, including sponge rubber, soft rubber, dense cotton, and molded materials. Try several noise protectors to find the one most comfortable for you—so you will wear it. If your ears ring after noise exposure while wearing a noise defender, change the type of defender you are using or wear an ear muff.

When around very loud noises, ear muffs are the only defender that will protect your ears. Ear muffs also vary in type. Under rare circumstances, both an ear canal noise defender and an ear muff must be worn to protect the ears.

Government regulations exist in the workplace that make it mandatory to use ear protection. But equally loud noises exist in the home and with hobbies. If you hear loud noises that hurt your ears, cause ringing, or cause you to shout to be heard—wear a noise defender!

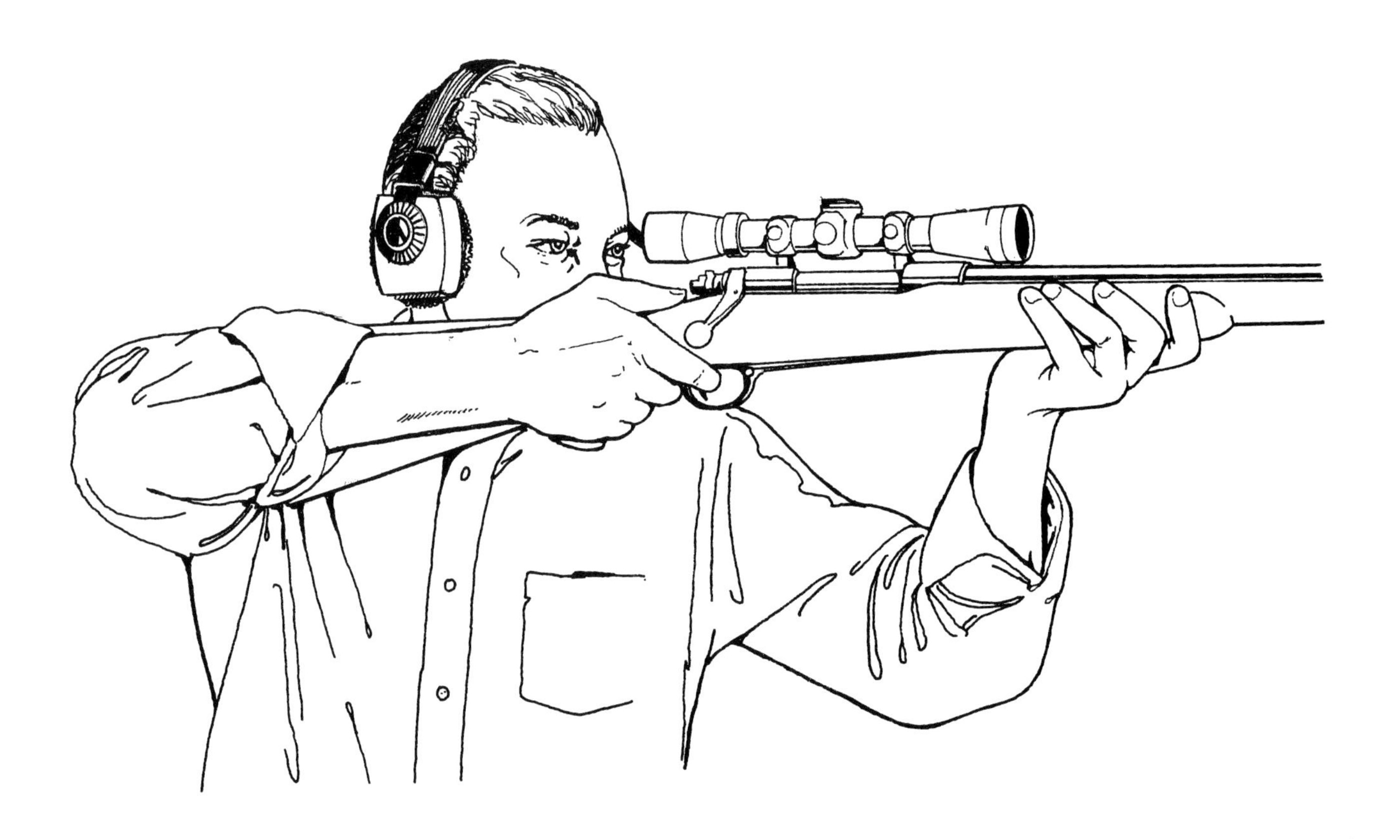

What Is a Diabetic Diet?

Good diabetes control means keeping your blood-sugar level as close to normal as possible. You need to maintain a proper balance between the insulin you produce or receive in a shot and the sugar your body makes out of the food you eat. You should maintain a nutritious, healthy diet that would be good for anyone. The main differences are that your diet contains limited or no added sugar that could raise blood-sugar levels too high, specifies the amount of food to be eaten, and sets specific times to eat for regulatory purposes. You should also maintain a proper weight.

What should I eat?

Eat foods from the six main food groups—milk, meat, vegetables, breads, fats, and fruits. Most diabetic meal plans list foods in terms of exchanges. Exchanges are units of measure that help you keep calories and types of foods controlled but allow variety by letting you trade one exchange for another food in the same group. Within each food group, serving sizes are adjusted to provide about the same amount of calories, carbohydrates, protein, and fat.

Isn't fat bad for you? Why can I eat fruits but not sugars?

Fat is a nutrient, and you need some fat in your diet. But too much fat can be harmful for people with diabetes because it increases the risk of heart disease and hardening of the arteries. Follow these tips:

- Avoid "hidden" fat (e.g., creamy pasta sauces, gravies), fried foods, and high-fat salad dressings.
- Choose lean meats; eat more fish and skinned poultry. Eat liver or organ meats only occasionally.
- Use diet margarine instead of butter.
- Drink lowfat or nonfat milk.
- Limit intake of eggs to 2 or 3 a week.

People with diabetes should eat less sugar. Depending on your individualized plan, some fruits may be encouraged because they provide fiber and carbohydrates for energy.

What foods should I stay away from?

Besides monitoring your intake of fats and sugars, you may need to restrict your intake of salt too. You should avoid other "ready sweets" like candy, jam, jelly, syrup, most cakes, pies and pastries, regular soda, jello, condensed milk, and sweet pickles.

What about packaged foods?

Learn to read and understand food labels. A *dietetic* label does not necessarily mean that the product is intended for diabetics. Labels list food ingredients in the order of relative quantity. Check food labels of all products. Avoid those that contain hidden sugars such as sucrose, mannitol, glucose, sorbitol, fructose, dextrose, corn syrup, invert sugar, and lactose. Consult your doctor or nutritional counselor before buying foods that are labeled *fat free.*

You can still enjoy eating out at restaurants. Choose restaurants that are sensitive to the current public interest in fitness and nutrition. Here are a few ideas to keep your blood sugar under control:

- Order fruits as either a dessert or an appetizer.
- Ask for your salad dressing "on the side" so that you can control the portion.
- Make sure your meat or fish course is broiled, baked, roasted, or poached—*never* fried!
- Avoid foods that may have unknown ingredients (e.g., foods with sauces).
- Ask how your food will be prepared.
- Some fast food restaurants can give you written information about their ingredients and are written with diabetic concerns in mind. The American Diabetes Association can also provide information.

What about alcohol?

Talk to your doctor before drinking alcohol. If your doctor says you may drink some alcohol, you will most likely *only* be able to have one or two alcoholic drinks, 1 or 2 times a week. The drink can be either a mixed drink with 1 ½ oz of alcohol, 4 oz of dry wine, or 12 oz of light beer. If you have type I diabetes, eat before you drink any alcohol to avoid low blood sugar and hypoglycemia. Alcohol interferes with glucose production in the liver, which is the glucose used by the body during an episode of hypoglycemia. Even if you eat, hypoglycemia can still occur several hours later, so follow your meal plan and check your blood sugar. Alcohol does have calories.

Do not add fruit juice or sweetened mixers to alcohol; use diet soft drinks, club soda, seltzer, and water. Avoid drinks containing sugars or starches, such as beer and sweet wines.

Alcohol can also cause low blood sugar in some people with type II diabetes who take oral medications. The combination of medication and alcohol may cause flushed skin in some people.

It is all right to cook with alcohol. When alcohol is heated, most of the alcohol evaporates. This leaves few calories but adds flavor to the food in which it is cooked.

How will other medications affect my alcohol intake?

You must check with your doctor about how alcohol may affect other medication you are taking. Remember too that your judgment and control will be impaired after a few drinks. You may forget an injection, forget to eat, or eat too much. To be safe, follow these tips:

- Before you start drinking, decide how much you will eat and drink.
- Put less alcohol in your mixed drinks.
- Drink slowly; make one drink last.
- Do *not* drink and drive.

Exercise and Diabetes

What does exercise have to do with my diabetes?

Exercise provides several benefits. Perhaps the most significant benefit to diabetes is that it usually lowers blood sugar and helps your body better use its food supply. Good diabetes control means keeping your blood-sugar level as close as possible to normal (between 90 and 140 mg/dL). Exercise may also help insulin work better. And exercise can lower cholesterol and triglyceride levels.

Exercise also improves the blood flow through small blood vessels, increases the heart's ability to pump, helps burn excess calories, and relieves tension, anxiety, and depression. If you are overweight (9 out of 10 people with type II diabetes are), an exercise diet plan can help you lose weight.

Your health care provider is in the best position to help you decide when you should exercise and what kind and how much exercise is best for you. Even after you begin an exercise regimen, you should not exercise if your blood-sugar control is poor. You and your doctor will reevaluate your exercise needs if you develop retinopathy or blood vessel problems.

How do I begin exercising?

The next step is to select an exercise regimen that would be fun for you. Begin gradually and increase your workout time. Your goal will be to exercise a minimum of 20 to 30 minutes and a maximum of 45 to 60 minutes at least 3 or 4 times per week. Be consistent and exercise at the same time and same intensity every day. A good time to exercise is 15 to 30 minutes after a meal, when the blood-sugar level is elevated. Do not exercise strenuously in the late evening, since your blood sugar continues to fall hours after completing your exercise.

Besides consistency, what else should my exercise program contain?

Every exercise program should have warm-up and a cool-down time to slowly stretch and "warm up" the muscles and then to slowly decrease the intensity and speed before stopping completely. *Never* skip the warm-up and cool-down periods. Take your pulse before starting any exercise program and retake your pulse before and after cool down. Your pulse should have increased before cool down and decreased after it. Your doctor will help you determine your target heart rates and show you how to take your pulse.

Are there special precautions for people with insulin-dependent (type I) diabetes?

First, consult your doctor. Plan your activity to fit in with your meal plan and with the action times and amounts of your insulin. Avoid exercise when blood sugar is consistently high and ketones are present in the urine. Also, avoid exercise at peak action time. For short-acting insulin, this peak action time would be 2 to 4 hours after injection; for intermediate- acting insulin, this would be 6 to 12 hours after injection.

In addition, never inject insulin into parts of your body that you use during exercise because insulin would be absorbed into the bloodstream too quickly. If you jog, do not inject insulin into your legs; if you weight-lift or play tennis, stay away from sites in the arms and legs.

It is wise to check your blood-sugar level before you begin exercising. If your blood-sugar level is low or in a normal range, you need a snack before starting so that you prevent an insulin reaction. Remember, an insulin reaction is characterized by feelings of hunger, faintness, sweating, dizziness, and confusion. An insulin reaction can occur while you exercise or up to 12 hours later.

In fact, regardless of your blood-sugar level, you should eat within an hour of exercising. If you do not eat a full meal, then eat a high-carbohydrate snack, such as 6 oz of fruit juice or half a bagel before light to moderate exercise (e.g., walking, biking, golf). If you plan to do heavier exercise (e.g., aerobics, running, squash, handball), you may need to eat a little more, such as half a meat sandwich and a cup of lowfat milk.

These precautions will minimize the possibility of an insulin reaction, but there are no guarantees. That is why it is a good idea not to exercise alone if you can prevent it. If you exercise with others, let somebody know that you have diabetes and teach that person how to help you. If you prefer running or cycling, ask a friend or relative to go with you. If you cannot find anyone to go with you, let someone know where you are going and when you'll be back.

What should I do if I do start to have an insulin reaction?

Stop exercising *immediately* and drink a half cup of orange juice or nondiet soft drink or take three glucose tablets right away. Treat an insulin reaction as soon as you feel it. Do not wait, or it may become worse. Whenever you exercise, *always* bring along raisins or hard candy just in case you need to raise your blood-sugar level.

Are there special precautions for people with non–insulin-dependent (type II) diabetes?

Exercise is particularly important for people with type II diabetes, since diet and exercise are the two keys to controlling diabetes for many of them. Exercise helps lower blood-sugar levels. Exercise burns calories that would otherwise be stored as excess weight. Exercise is a valuable tool for preventing heart disease.

Always check with your doctor before starting any exercise program, especially because you do run a higher risk for heart disease. If you use insulin or oral diabetes medication, you should know your blood-sugar level before you start exercising. If you are low, you will need a snack before you begin.

Good Foot Care

Take Care of Your Feet

Every day the average person takes about 10,000 steps and during a lifetime you may walk 115,000 miles. This is equal to walking around the earth 4 ½ times. Every step you take exerts a force that is greater than your body weight. The force goes directly to your feet and causes a pounding wear-and-tear on the bones and muscles of the feet.

Common Foot Problems

Part of caring for your feet includes early recognition of common foot problems. Do not let problems with your feet go untreated; consult a health care provider for proper care.

- ***Bunions*** are deformities of the bone joints of the big toe that cause the first joint to slant outward and often rub against the shoe. This, in turn, may lead to irritation, swelling, and redness.
- ***Calluses and corns*** are thickening of the skin. A callus is a thickened pad of skin, usually on the weight-bearing part of the sole of the foot. A corn is a callus with a painful core that occurs at a pressure point such as the top of the toe or under the joint of the toe. Either may become painful.
- ***Hammertoe*** is a permanently bent, clawlike deformity of the middle joint of the toe. The toe bends up and then bends down. If the toe rubs against the shoe, it may become inflamed and sore.
- ***Heel pain*** may be caused by a *heel spur* (a hook of bony growth at the bottom of the heel bone), *plantar fasciitis* (inflammation of a band of tissue that connects the heel bone to the toes), or *bruising* of the heel bone from walking on a hard surface.
- ***Plantar warts*** are viral lesions *(caused by Papilloma virus)* that may appear on the sole of the foot. They may be contagious, are painful, and make walking difficult.
- ***Athlete's foot*** is a fungal infection of the foot that causes scaliness and cracking of the skin between the toes and on the soles of the feet. Athlete's foot may spread to other parts of the body, especially the hands. It is contagious and frequently recurs.
- ***Ingrown toenail*** is a toenail edge that curves into the skin on the side of the toe. This may cause redness, swelling, and pain.

How to Prevent Feet Problems

In addition to recognizing common problems, there are many things that you can do to promote healthy feet and prevent problems. Follow these guidelines:

- Walk regularly. This will improve circulation, increase flexibility, and encourage bone and muscle development. Walking is very important for maintaining overall foot health.
- Always wear comfortable shoes that provide proper support. The shoes should be sufficiently wide and have low enough heels so that you feel no leg fatigue, leg or foot cramps, or pain.
- Massage your feet to improve circulation and promote relaxation of the feet at least daily.
- If you have bunions, wear shoes that are extra long or wide. This will help ease pressure on your toes. In addition, use donut-shaped bunion cushions or mole-skin to take pressure off of the joints.
- Wear heel pads or cushions in the bottom of your shoes to protect your heels if you walk on hard surfaces for long times.
- Wash your feet every day in warm water. Dry them by blotting with a towel, rather than rubbing.
- If your feet perspire a lot, dust your feet with talc or a hygienic foot powder. You may also sprinkle some powder into your shoes. Do not use cornstarch powder because it may lead to a fungal infection.
- Trim your nails shortly after you have taken a bath or shower, while they are soft. Cut the nails straight across with a toenail clipper.
- Do not go barefoot outdoors, especially if you are in an area that is not your own yard. A foreign body may cut or puncture your foot.
- Inspect your feet every day for cuts, blisters, and scratches. Provide care as needed and observe for proper healing.

If You Have Diabetes

Foot care takes on a special importance if you have diabetes. Because of possible circulatory and neurologic problems that may occur in people with diabetes, it is important that you pay attention to your feet. Note and report any of the following to your health care provider:

- A persistent sensation of cold, numbness, tingling, or burning sensation in the feet or legs
- Discoloration of the skin (either pale or dark), loss of hair on the legs, or muscle cramps or tightness
- Any sign of a foot infection, ulcer, or open wound on the foot that does not heal quickly.

Healthy feet are crucial for an active and independent lifestyle. Foot problems and foot pain are not normal. Regardless of how old you are, it is important that you take care of your feet.

Prevention, Screening, and Early Detection of Cancer

The number of people who develop cancer is on the rise—it is estimated that one in three Americans will have some type of cancer. Some of these cancers can be cured in the early stages, but not when the disease is too advanced. Early detection and treatment are the keys to curing cancer; preventing cancer in the first place is even better.

General prevention guidelines

There is much you can do help prevent cancer. Smoking has been scientifically proven to cause cancer, so if you smoke, stop. What you eat can also have an effect on whether you develop cancer. The following are dietary recommendations for preventing cancer:

- Reduce the amount of fat in your diet to 30% of your total daily calorie intake.
- Limit the amount of alcohol you drink to one or two drinks a day.
- Limit the amount of charbroiled, smoked, and salted foods you eat.
- Maintain your ideal weight.
- Eat foods high in:
  - Vitamin A—apricots, peaches, carrots, spinach, asparagus, squash, and sweet potatoes
  - Vitamin C—oranges, lemons, grapefruit, strawberries, tomatoes, cabbage, and walnuts
  - Vitamin E—lettuce, alfalfa, and vegetable oils
  - Fiber—fresh vegetables and fruits, whole grain breads and cereals, nuts, beans, and peas

Prevention, screening, and early detection guidelines for common cancers

Breast Cancer. Reduce the amount of fat in your diet. Any one or a combination of these signs may be a warning signal for cancer: a lump in the breast; dimpling of the skin; a sinking in of the nipple, or discharge from the nipple; swelling in the breast; or a change in the size or shape of the breast. Early detection includes breast self-examination once a month; a yearly breast examination by a health care provider; a baseline mammogram between the ages of 35 and 39; and a yearly mammogram after age 40. If you have a family history of breast cancer, you should start having mammograms at age 30.*

Cervical Cancer. Avoid sex at an early age (especially before age 18), and do not have numerous partners. Use condoms, and practice good perineal hygiene. Cancer warning signs include abnormal vaginal bleeding and spotting after having sex. Early detection involves an annual Pap smear for women over age 18. After at least three normal examinations, the test can be done less often.

Colon/Rectal Cancer. Follow the dietary guidelines listed above. Have colorectal polyps removed. Cancer warning signs include rectal bleeding, a change in stools, pain in the abdomen, and pressure on the rectum. Early detection includes an annual digital rectal examination starting at age 40; an annual stool blood test starting at age 50; and an annual inspection of the colon with a special instrument (sigmoidoscopy) starting at age 50.

Endometrial Cancer. Follow the dietary guidelines listed above. Discuss with your doctor the benefits and risks of estrogen therapy if you are past menopause. Cancer warning signs include abnormal vaginal bleeding and pain or a mass in the abdomen. Early detection includes pelvic examinations and endometrial biopsy at menopause and in high-risk women.

Head and Neck Cancer. Follow the dietary guidelines listed above. Avoid tobacco in all forms. Practice good oral hygiene. Cancer warning signs include difficulty chewing; a persistent sore throat; hoarseness; a color change in the mouth; earache; a lump in the neck; loss of sense of smell; and difficulty breathing. Early detection includes monthly oral self-examination and an annual physical exam.

Lung Cancer. Do not smoke. Follow guidelines at work to reduce exposure to cancer-causing substances. Warning signs include a persistent cough or cold; pain in the chest; wheezing; difficulty breathing; and a change in the volume or odor of phlegm. No tests exist for early detection.

Prostate Cancer. There are no prevention guidelines for prostate cancer. Warning signs include difficulty urinating, painful and frequent urination, and blood in the urine. Early detection includes an annual digital rectal exam starting at age 40; measurement of PSA is controversial.

Skin Cancer. Use a sunscreen with a sun protection factor (SPF) of at least 15 (the SPF is shown on the bottle), and wear protective clothing when in the sun. Avoid tanning booths. Cancer warning signs include a change in a wart or mole, and a sore that does not heal. Early detection includes an annual physical examination, monthly self-examination of the skin, and paying particular attention to moles, warts, and birthmarks.

Testicular Cancer. No prevention guidelines exist for testicular cancer. Cancer warning signs include swelling, a lump, or a heavy feeling in the testicle. Early detection includes an annual physical exam and monthly testicular self-exam.

*American Cancer Society guidelines; National Cancer Institute recommends baseline mammogram at or about age 50 for women not at risk.

Sun Exposure Risks

A beautiful suntan may get you smiles, but it is no longer considered a sign of healthy skin. Exposure to the sun is a causative factor of the more than 600,000 new cases of skin cancer that are diagnosed in the United States each year. At highest risk for these cancers are fair-skinned individuals, Caucasians in particular, who have a long history of exposure to the sun. This includes people who began long periods of sun exposure during childhood and adolescence, as well as adults who spend their working or leisure time outdoors in the sun. Because of the protective melanin in the skin, African-Americans and people from other dark-skinned races are less likely to acquire skin cancer.

The good news is that many skin cancers are preventable. The prevention includes protecting your skin with clothing and the use of sunscreens from exposure to the sun.

Sunscreens

When it is not possible to avoid exposure to the sun, sunscreens may be used to develop a protective layer between the ultraviolet rays of the sun and the skin. The choice of sunscreen should be based on your skin type, the length of time you spend in the sun, the intensity of the sun's rays where you are, and the type of sunscreen you prefer. The Food and Drug Administration designates five categories of protection that have been scored according to the amount of their sun protection factor (SPF). The higher the SPF, the greater the protection against the sun's ultraviolet rays. Products with SPF 15 or greater provide the greatest protection against sun-induced skin damage and against sun-caused skin cancers.

SUNSCREENS
SUN PROTECTION FACTOR (SPF)

SPF 2 to 4	Minimal sun protection
SPF 4 to 6	Moderate sun protection
SPF 6 to 8	Extra sun protection
SPF 8 to 15	Maximum sun protection
SPF 15 to greater	Ultra sun protection

Many sunscreens also contain chemicals that protect against the sun's rays (particularly UV-B, which are the familiar sunburn and skin cancer causing rays). These chemicals are PABA, PABA esters, and cinnamates. When the sunscreens are combined with one of these chemicals, they provide the maximum protection against the sun's rays.

Sun Protection Techniques

There are many things you can do to protect your skin from the ultraviolet rays of the sun. These include such things as the following:

- ♦ Limit your sun exposure during the midday hours (10:00 AM to 3:00 PM) when the sun is the strongest.
- ♦ Plan outdoor activities, such as walking and gardening, for early morning or late afternoon.
- ♦ Wear protective clothing such as a wide-brimmed hat, a long-sleeved shirt, and long pants when in the sun.
- ♦ Use a sunscreen with a sun protection factor (SPF) of 15 or higher when exposed to the sun. The sunscreen should be applied 15 to 30 minutes before going into the sunlight and every 2 to 3 hours during exposure (it may need to be applied more often because of heat, humidity, and sweating). If one sunscreen irritates your skin, try another; there are dozens of good ones.
- ♦ Use a sunscreen when participating in high-altitude activities like mountain climbing and skiing. At high altitudes the exposure to ultraviolet rays is greatest. The sun is also stronger near the equator.
- ♦ Use a sunscreen even on overcast days. The sun's rays can still be damaging when filtered through clouds.
- ♦ Avoid sun exposure if you are taking a medication that causes *photosensitivity* (an increased sensitivity of the skin to sunburn). Examples of these medications include diuretics, antihistamines, antidepressants, antibiotics, and oral hypoglycemics. Consult your health care provider to determine if your medication may cause photosensitivity.
- ♦ Avoid tanning booths. The ultraviolet light in tanning booths is as risky as that from the sun.
- ♦ Be aware of the reflective surfaces such as sand, snow, concrete, and water. Sitting near these surfaces, even if you are in the shade, increases your exposure to the sun's rays.
- ♦ Keep infants out of the sun. Begin using sunscreens as early as 6 months of age.
- ♦ Teach children about sun protection at an early age. Children should be taught to protect themselves from the sun because sun damage accumulates over a lifetime.

Warning: Squamous and Basal Cell Cancer

Skin cancer is the most common type of cancer found in humans. Each year over 600,000 new cases of skin cancer are diagnosed. Squamous cell and basal cell carcinoma (cancer) are the two most common types of skin cancer found among people with light or fair skin, light hair, and blue, green, or gray eyes. Both basal cell and squamous cell carcinomas are more frequently found in men than women. Basal cell carcinoma is most commonly found in men 40 years and older and squamous cell skin cancer is most commonly found in men 60 years and older. Persons at highest risk for developing skin cancer are those whose occupations or recreation expose them to the sun. Examples include: mariners, farmers, outdoor construction workers, swimmers, golfers, and other outdoor athletes.

Signs of Squamous Cell Cancer

Squamous cell carcinoma appears as a scaly, slightly elevated lesion (sore). Often the lesion may have a crater or ulcerated center. It is frequently found on the back of the hands and forearm, as well as on the head and neck (especially on the ears, lower lip, scalp, and forehead). It is found most often on areas of the skin where there has been previous sun-damage or sunburn.

The cure rate for squamous cell carcinoma is 75% to 80% when it is treated with surgery or radiation therapy. If left untreated, squamous cell carcinoma can metastasize to the lymph nodes and/or to other body systems.

Signs of Basal Cell Cancer

Basal cell carcinoma often appears as a single, small, firm, dome-shaped, flesh-colored nodule. It has raised edges and a pearly white border. Small red vessels may be seen in thin skin areas. The lesion is often described as a pimple that has not healed, with an ulcerated bleeding center. The most common location for basal cell cancer is on the face, especially the cheeks, forehead, eyelids, and folds around the nose.

If identified and promptly treated by surgical excision or radiation, 90% to 95% of all patients are considered cured. If left untreated, the tumor will invade such vital structures as blood vessels, lymph nodes, nerves, cartilage, bones, and other body systems.

Protecting Your Skin

The skin's exposure to the sun and environmental irritants (such as coal, tar, creosote, arsenic compounds, and radium) are the major risk factors for developing both basal cell and squamous cell cancers. The sun alone causes at least 90% of all skin cancers. You may protect yourself from the sun and other exposures by observing the following:

- Avoid intense sunlight between 10:00 AM and 3:00 PM, when the ultraviolet rays are the strongest.
- Plan outdoor activities such as walking, gardening, and other hobbies for early morning or late afternoon.
- Wear protective clothing such as a wide-brimmed hat and a long-sleeved shirt when either in the sun or near environmental exposure to irritants.
- Use a sunscreen with a sun protection factor (SPF) of 15 or higher when in the sun. The sunscreen should be applied 15 to 30 minutes before going into the sunlight and every 2 to 3 hours during exposure (it may need to be applied more often because of heat, humidity, and sweating).
- Avoid tanning booths.
- Wash your skin as soon as possible following skin contamination from coal, tar, creosote, arsenic compounds, or radium.

Examining Your Skin

Most often you will be the one to identify a malignant change on your own skin. Most frequently this will be a change in a wart or mole or a sore that does not heal. You should examine your skin each month and report any changes to your health care provider. Particular attention should be paid to moles, warts, and birthmarks. Check with your health care provider for instructions on how to perform a proper self-examination of the skin.

Skin Self-Examination

The number of cases of skin cancer is on the rise. Steps for preventing skin cancer include wearing a sunscreen with a high sun protection factor (SPF 15 or higher); staying out of the midday sun, if possible; and performing a monthly skin self-examination.

Examining your skin once a month can help you detect any moles, blemishes, or birthmarks that have changed in size, shape, or color, or a sore that does not heal. If you find any of these signs, see your doctor at once.

How to do skin self-examination

You will need a hand mirror and a full-length mirror to examine yourself.

1. Using a full-length mirror, examine the front and back of your body. Then raise your arms and examine the sides of your body (Figure 1).
2. Check the skin under your forearms and upper arms and on the palms of your hands.
3. Sit down and look at the backs of your legs. Examine your feet, including the soles and between your toes (Figure 2).
4. Examine the back of your neck and your scalp with a hand mirror (Figure 3).

Examining your skin once a month will help you familiarize yourself with the normal appearance of your skin. It is also a good idea to visit a dermatologist once a year for a thorough skin examination.

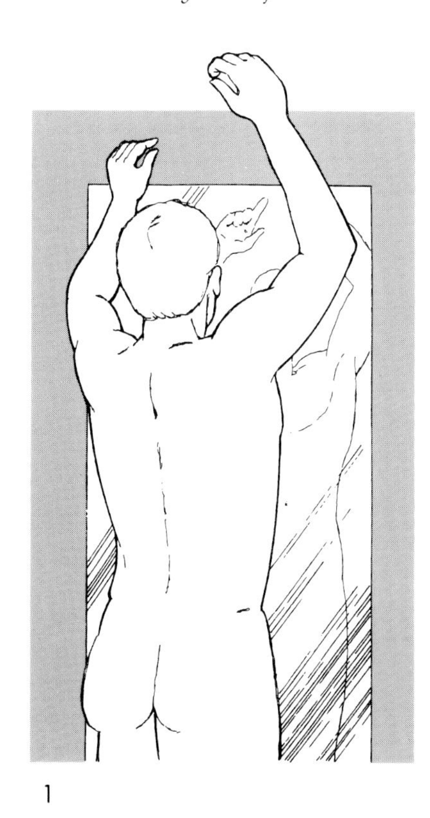

1

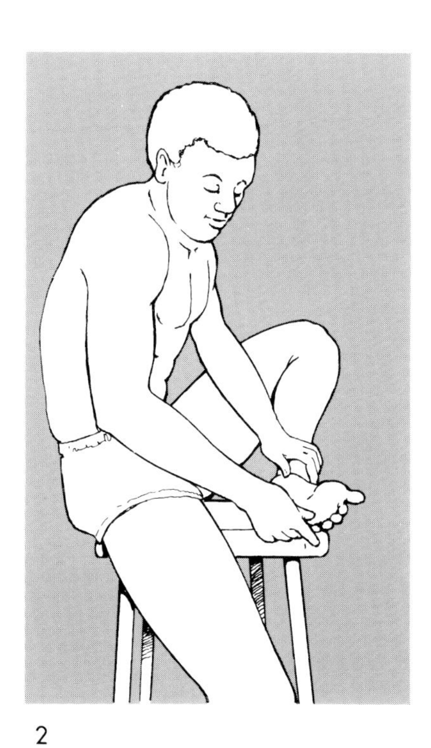

2

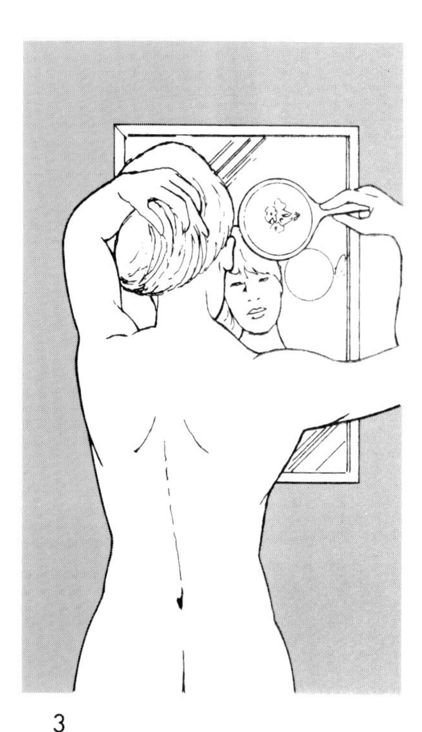

3

Breast Self-Examination

Performing breast self-examination once a month could save your life. Many breast cancers are discovered by patients who had regularly done self-exam and thus were able to distinguish a change from what is normal in their breasts. If you are still menstruating, examine your breasts right after your period ends. If you have reached menopause, pick a day of the month that is easy to remember.

How to do breast self-examination

1. Undress and stand in front of a mirror with your arms at your sides. Look for any changes in the shape or size of your breasts or anything unusual, such as discharge from the nipples or puckering or dimpling of the skin (Figure 1).
2. Raise your arms above and behind your head, and press your hands together. Look for the same things as in step 1 (Figure 2).
3. Place the palms of your hands firmly on your hips; look again for any changes (Figure 3).
4. Raise your left arm over your head. Examine your left breast by firmly pressing the fingers of your right hand down and around in a circular motion until you have examined every part of the breast. You may use the wedge section, circular, or vertical strip examination method.* Be sure to include the area between your breast and armpit and the armpit itself. You are feeling for any lump or mass under the skin. If you find a lump, notify your doctor (Figure 4).
5. Gently squeeze the nipple, and look for any discharge (Figure 5). If there is any, see your doctor.
6. Repeat steps 4 and 5 on your right breast. (You may also perform steps 4 and 5 in the shower.)
7. Now, lie down on your back with a pillow under your right shoulder. Put your right arm over your head (Figure 6). This position flattens the breast and makes it easier to examine. Examine your right breast just as you did in steps 4 and 5. Repeat on your left breast.

Do not panic if you notice anything unusual. This does not necessarily mean you have cancer. Notify your doctor and let him or her examine you. *Remember: Breast self-examination is important, but it is not a substitute for a doctor's examination and regular mammograms for women over age 40.*

*Ask your doctor for information on the various breast exam methods.

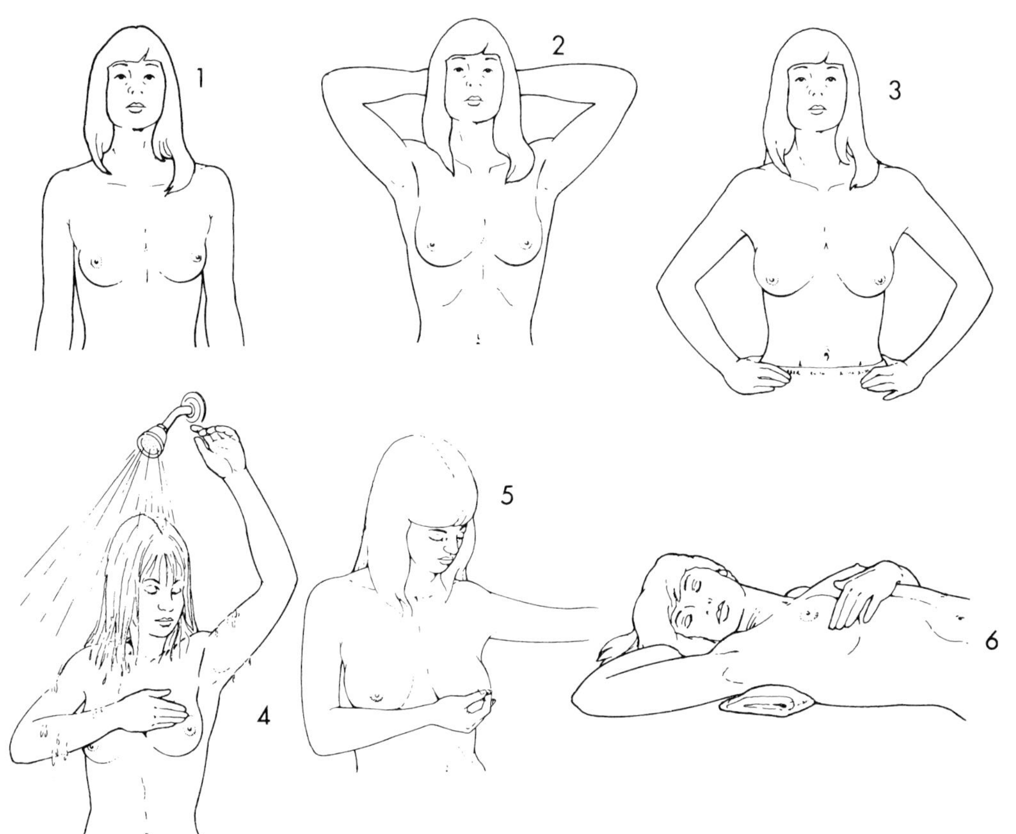

Vulvar Self-Examination

Cancer of the vulva is still a rare disease, but it is occurring more frequently. Women over age 50 are most susceptible to this cancer, but it can occur at any age. Examining your vulvar area once a month can help you discover the first symptoms of vulvar cancer, which can be cured if treated early. The vulvar area includes all the female external genital organs: the pubic mound, clitoris, urinary opening, vaginal opening, and anus (Figure 1).

How to do vulvar self-examination

Use a flashlight and a hand mirror to make viewing easier. You may do the examination while sitting on the edge of the toilet seat, your bed, or the bathtub. Sit with your legs spread apart, and check the entire vulvar region (Figure 2).

Examine both sides of the labia (the opening folds of the vulva), and see if they are similar.

With your fingers, separate the inner lips of the vulva, and check the clitoris, the urinary opening, the vagina, and the skin between the vagina and anus (Figure 3).

Press down on all areas of the vulva, feeling for any lumps or masses (Figure 4).

Gently squeeze the vaginal opening between your thumb and forefinger. It should feel soft and moist (not be tender or sore) (Figure 5).

If you see any of the following, see your doctor:

- Lumps, masses, or growths
- Any change in skin color
- Moles or birthmarks on the vulva that change color, bleed, or enlarge
- Burning in the vulva during urination
- Persistent itching
- Soreness or tenderness that does not go away
- Usually these signs do not indicate cancer, but check with your doctor to make sure.

What causes vulvar cancer, and what can I do to prevent it?

It is unclear what causes cancer in the vulvar area, but certain conditions are thought to lead to the disease. These include poor hygiene, certain types of sexually transmitted diseases, cancer of other reproductive organs, and a condition called dystrophy, in which the skin of the vulva may thin or thicken, and red or white patches and sores may appear. You can help prevent some of these problems by seeing your gynecologist at least once a year, reporting any changes you find during your vulvar self-examination, and practicing good hygiene. Good hygiene of the vulva includes the following:

- Wiping from front to back after urination or a bowel movement
- Avoiding scented and perfumed products such as tampons, sanitary pads, feminine hygiene products, and scented soaps
- Using unscented, white toilet paper
- Wearing all-cotton underwear
- Avoiding tight clothing such as girdles, pantyhose, and form-fitting jeans

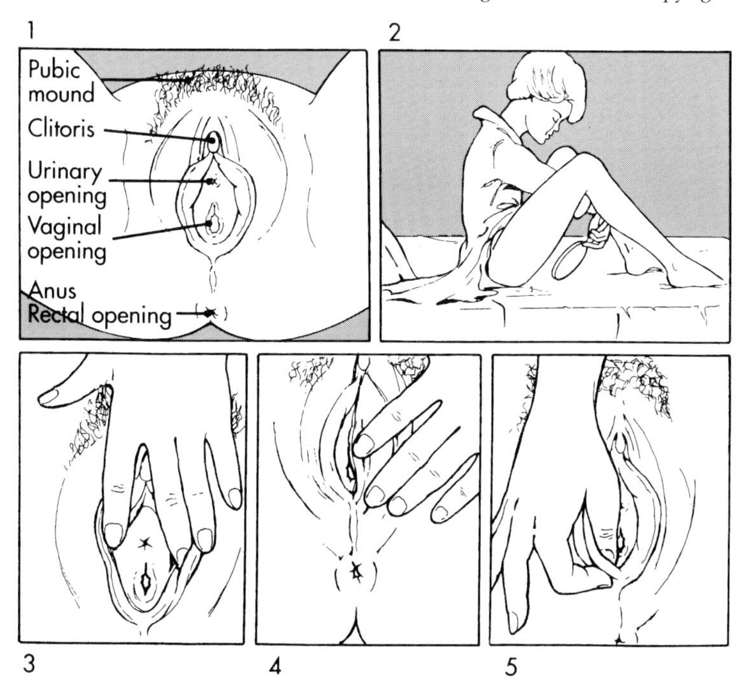

Testicular Self-Examination

Testicular cancer is a curable disease if it is discovered and treated early. Performing testicular self-examination (TSE) once a month greatly increases the chances that you will discover a cancerous lump or mass early enough for effective treatment.

When you do testicular self-examination you should be looking for hard nodules or lumps in the testes. Enlarged testes also may indicate a cancerous condition, and any enlargement or swelling that doesn't respond to medications should be investigated further.

How to do testicular self-examination

Boys should begin examining themselves at 15 years of age and should perform the examination once a month. Choose a day of the month that is significant to you, such as your birthday or the first or fifteenth of the month, to make it easier for you to remember to do the examination regularly.

It is best to examine the testicles in a warm place, such as the shower, because this promotes relaxation and descent of the scrotal contents. Soap your hands to increase your sensitivity to touch. Use both hands during the examination.

1. Examine each testicle separately; apply only gentle pressure while holding the scrotum in your palm. The testicles should be approximately equal in size and evenly round. No nodules should be present.
2. Examine your right testicle first. Lift your penis with your left hand, and with your right hand locate the epididymis, the cordlike structure at the back of your testicle. Feel along it with your thumb and first two fingers. The epididymis extends upward into the spermatic cord. Squeeze gently along the length of this cord, feeling for lumps and masses as you progress upward. It normally is tender to the touch.
3. Identify the vas deferens. It is a smooth, movable tube that can be traced up to the point where the scrotum joins the groin. It should be movable, nontender, and of equal size in the two testicles.
4. Repeat steps 2 and 3 to examine the left testicle, using your left hand.

Normal testicles should feel firm to the touch, but you should be able to move them. They should feel smooth and rubbery and should be free of lumps. If you notice any lumps or masses or anything unusual, call your doctor.

Know the signs of testicular cancer. They are:

- A change in the size or consistency of one testicle
- A lump or nodule on one testicle
- Pain or a sensation of testicular pressure or heaviness
- Enlargement of your nipples

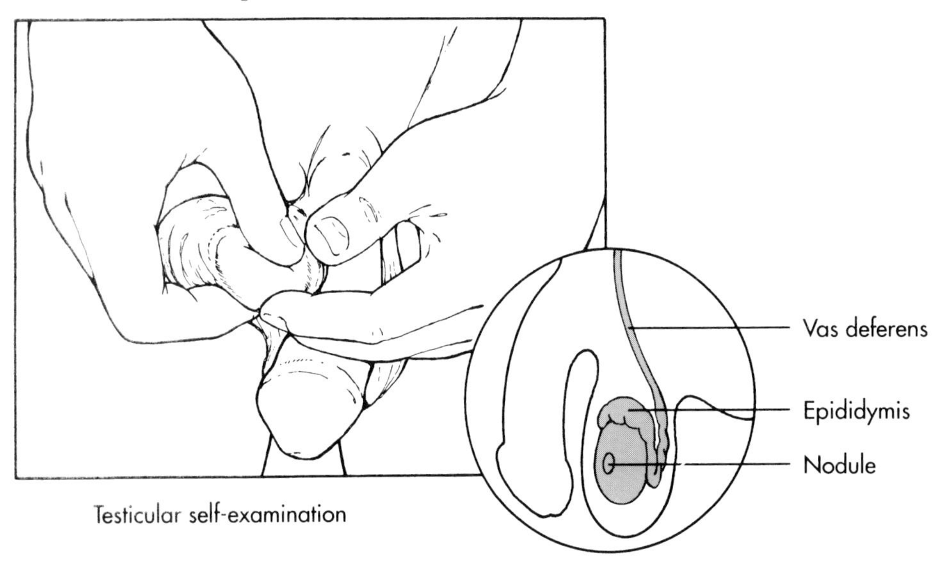

Testicular self-examination

Safer Sex

What does it mean to practice "safer sex"?

The term "safer sex" refers to the practice of protecting yourself against sexually transmitted diseases (STDs), sometimes referred to as venereal disease (VD). There are at least 50 different kinds of these diseases, some of them even life-threatening. You can catch an STD by having sex with someone who is infected.

What if I have sex without actually having intercourse?

You can still get an STD without having vaginal intercourse or penetration. STDs are spread by having vaginal, oral, or anal sex with an infected person. STD-causing germs can pass from one person to another through body fluids such as semen, vaginal fluid, saliva, and blood; genital warts and herpes are STDs that are spread by direct contact with a wart or blister.

No one I date looks to me as if they could have an STD. They look really healthy.

You can't tell if a person has an STD just by appearance. In fact, some people with STDs have no signs at all and may not even know they are infected. Still, some signs to look for in your partner are a heavy discharge, rash, sore, or redness near your partner's sex organs. If you see any of these, don't have sex or be sure to use a condom.

How can I tell if I might have an STD?

You may have an STD if you experience burning or pain when urinating; sores, bumps, or blisters near the genitals or mouth; swelling around the genitals; fever, chills, night sweats, or swollen glands; or tiredness, vomiting, diarrhea, or sore muscles. In addition, you may have an unusual discharge or smell from the vagina; burning and itching around the vagina; pain in the lower abdomen; vaginal pain during sex; or vaginal bleeding between periods. *But don't forget; you may not have any warning signs at all. Regular medical checkups are essential to your health. If you have sex with more than one partner, routine cultures and blood tests may be needed.*

I think I have an STD! What should I do?

Get help right away. If you don't, you may pass the STD to your partner or, if you're pregnant, to your baby. In fact, without treatment an STD may make it impossible for you to have a baby at all. You may also develop brain damage, blindness, cancer, heart disease, or arthritis. In some cases you can even die. So go to a doctor or clinic right away.

If your health care provider determines that you do have an STD, tell your partner or partners to get tested, too. Take all of your medication; don't stop just because all your symptoms go away. Do not have sex until you have received full treatment. The disease could still be present in your body. Finally, keep all your appointments, and always use a condom and spermicide when you have sex.

What are the signs of STDs?

There are many different kinds of STDs, and some of them have similar symptoms. You should never attempt to make a diagnosis on your own. The nurse can give you a list with general descriptions of a few of the most common sexually transmitted diseases.

How can I reduce my chances of contracting an STD?

Remember, the more sexual partners you have, the greater your risk. Naturally, the best way to reduce your risk is by not having sex or by having sex with one mutually faithful, uninfected partner, or by using a latex condom and spermicide with nonoxynol 9 during sex. Some STDs may be avoided by placing spermicide in the vagina before having sex, because it kills sperm and some STD germs. It helps to urinate and wash after sex (but do not douche, because douching may actually force germs higher up into the body). Avoid having sex with someone who uses intravenous drugs or engages in anal sex. Don't engage in oral, anal, or vaginal sex with an infected person. If you think you may be at risk for AIDS or an STD, seek medical help immediately. Use a new condom each time you have sexual intercourse. *Recent research indicates that the prevention of HIV transmission and developing AIDS may be only 60% to 70% effective when using condoms as a barrier against this infection.*

What if the condom breaks? What should we do?

If a condom breaks, do not douche. Insert more spermicide into the vagina right away. Men should wash their genitals immediately. Go to a doctor or clinic for an STD examination as soon as possible.

Preventing Urinary Tract Infections

A urinary tract infection (UTI) is any infection or inflammation located along the urinary tract. Most urinary tract infections occur in the bladder or urethra, the canal that carries the urine from the bladder to the urethral opening.

What causes urinary tract infections?

Urinary tract infections have a number of causes. Most are caused by bacteria from the bowel that invade the urinary tract. Because a woman's urethra is closer to the rectum than a man's is, women suffer many more urinary tract infections than men do. Other causes include overstretching of the bladder, urine left in the bladder (incomplete voiding), and lack of cleanliness when doing catheterization. Urethral inflammation can be caused by chemical irritants such as perfumed feminine hygiene products, sanitary napkins, spermicidal foams and jellies, and bubble bath.

What are the signs of a urinary tract infection?

Several signs indicate a urinary tract infection. You may have one or a combination of these symptoms:

- A frequent and urgent need to urinate
- Pain in the lower back and lower pelvic region
- Cloudy, foul-smelling urine
- Blood urine
- Chills or fever
- Lack of appetite or lack of energy, or both
- Sandlike material (sediment) in the urine

How can I prevent a urinary tract infection or inflammation?

The most important thing you can do to prevent a urinary tract infection is to practice good hygiene. Women should avoid wiping fecal matter into the urethral area. Wiping from front to back helps prevent germs and bacteria from entering the urethral opening. Showering or bathing daily also helps prevent the spread of germs, and drinking lots of fluids helps the bladder flush itself.

If you are catheterizing yourself, it is very important that you are careful to be very clean. It is very easy to insert germs along with the catheter into your urethra and bladder. Wash your hands frequently as you carry out the catheterization process. Wash the catheter in soapy water after each use and allow it to dry completely before using it again.

To prevent inflammation of the urinary tract, avoid perfumed feminine hygiene products, spermicidal jellies and foams, and bubble bath.

See your doctor if you think you might have a urinary tract infection. Such infections can lead to bladder and kidney damage, kidney stones, and urine retention.

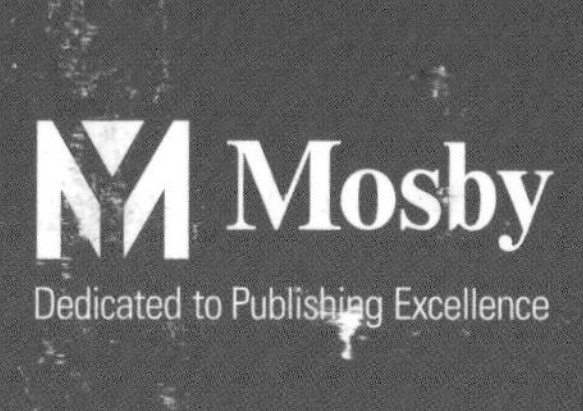

ISBN 0-8151-2574-7

31313